silent nights

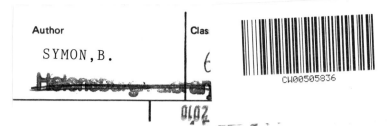

To my best friend

silent nights

Overcoming Sleep Problems in

Babies and Children

BRIAN SYMON

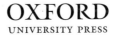
OXFORD
UNIVERSITY PRESS

OXFORD
UNIVERSITY PRESS

253 Normanby Road, South Melbourne, Victoria 3205, Australia

Oxford University Press is a department of the University of Oxford.
It furthers the University's objective of excellence in research, scholarship,
and education by publishing worldwide in

Oxford New York

Auckland Bangkok Buenos Aires Cape Town Chennai
Dar es Salaam Delhi Hong Kong Istanbul Karachi Kolkata
Kuala Lumpur Madrid Melbourne Mexico City Mumbai Nairobi
São Paulo Shanghai Taipei Tokyo Toronto

OXFORD is a trade mark of Oxford University Press
in the UK and in certain other countries

National Library of Australia
Cataloguing-in-Publication data:

Symon, B.
    Silent nights: overcoming sleep problems in babies
    and children

    Includes index.
    ISBN 0 19 551786 5.

    1. Infants—Sleep. 2. Children—Sleep. 3. Sleep
    Disorders in Children—Popular works. I. Title.

    649.122

Typeset by Solo Typesetting, South Australia
Printed through Bookpac Production Services, Singapore

Acknowledgments

While the writing of this book and its precursors has occurred over the space of probably fifteen years, there are some people who have had a great impact upon its development. I need to acknowledge the important contribution to my understanding of infants and young children played by my wife Maryanne. It is entirely due to her skill and wisdom with our own babies that I developed a special interest in the sleep of young children and babies. Her concepts led to my reading, researching, testing and experimenting. While I have been able to expand considerably on the analysis and study of sleep, this has simply confirmed many of the ideas which she initially presented to me. To our children Simon, Tim, Ben and Stephanie, thanks for your patience with my lifestyle. While a doctor's family are often left with the impression that they come last in terms of allocating time, the reverse is certainly the case in my heart.

Thank you to the hundreds of families who have been generous in placing faith in my ideas and allowed me to care for them in this special area.

I must also acknowledge those who have helped with reading, criticising, typing and retyping—in historical order Robyn, Christine, Paula, and finally my son Ben, who typed the final 20 000 words. Thank you all.

Contents

Introduction

This book is written in the belief that the early establishment of good sleep patterns in newborn infants is a major contribution to developing sanity and happiness for both the baby and her carers. It is also written in the belief, supported by experience, that a normal, healthy baby can learn good sleep patterns.

The book has grown out of notes I produced as an aid for my patients, first as a general practitioner in a country town and later as a city doctor with a special interest in the success of families with young children. It also draws on my own experience as a father of four children. More recently it has been used as a teaching tool in a research study to determine whether sleep performance of children in the first three months of life can be improved *before* there are any sleep problems. In these studies we were able to demonstrate improved sleep in the newborn infant by six weeks of age. This improvement was maintained at 12 weeks. The average improvement in sleep was nine hours of extra sleep per week compared to families who were not using the book or receiving the tutoring which went with it. (See Chapter 15 for more details of this study.)

In its original form the book was a guide for new parents and focused on the first few months of life. It now looks at the time from birth to some undefined time before school. Much of what is written applies to newborn children, but the oldest case I mention is ten years old.

I have written this book for the average couple. Take from it those pieces of advice which fit with your life and your beliefs. This is not a scientific book, but a collection of hints that I hope you will find useful.

Balance and harmony

How well we interact with others depends on the appropriateness of our behaviour. One code of behaviour exists at home, a modified code in another's home. One set of rules exists for one's children and a modified set for someone else's. As we grow older we recognise these differences more, and by becoming more flexible we interact more successfully and are more successful in our social circle.

The vast majority of people wish to live in harmony with others; to achieve a balance between privacy and satisfying our need for social interaction; to feel the security of receiving good leadership and the satisfaction of giving leadership to others; to feel a sense of belonging and at the same time to feel that your individuality is recognised; to give and receive love, both in reasonable measure.

It is the balance of these things, often contradictions, that produces harmony and contentment within our lives.

As parents, one of our aims is to help our children achieve harmony in their lives.

No stable house can be built on an unsound foundation. A rounded, stable individual is the result of a sound foundation at home. One of my aims in this book is to assist parents to begin work on producing a sound foundation for their children in the first weeks and years of life by finding a practical compromise in meeting contradictory needs.

The beginning of parenthood

The first weeks of a child's life are a time of challenge and intense learning for parents.

Pregnancy is a time of great expectations and of varying health. After months of waiting, labour begins. Labour varies dramatically in its ease or difficulty. The fortunate few have strong contractions for less than one hour and then deliver easily. After this they walk back to their rooms, smiling at the staff as they go. At the other extreme, an unfortunate few labour hard for more than 24 hours, require extensive pain relief, become exhausted, and finally have a difficult delivery or are assisted by forceps, caesarean or some other technique. These women take days to recuperate, and question why they ever planned to get pregnant and wonder how they might cope. The majority of mothers lie somewhere in between. Labour lasts between four and twelve hours, is handled with dignity, and results in the delivery of a healthy child from a tired but pleased mother.

While labour requires courage, strength, composure and cooperative effort, it is largely not a skill the mother has learned. By this I mean that the events of labour are largely determined by the body without conscious effort by the mother. Usually the body determines when labour starts, its rate of progress, and the details of the delivery. If the mother knows nothing about it, it will still happen. As long as she is attended by a companion, a midwife or an experienced medical attendant, then in the majority of occasions a live birth will occur.

Once the baby is born, however, the autopilot is off and learned skills are required. Advice from those providing care to the mother with a newborn child is very important, but that advice varies dramatically. When we have our first baby in our arms we receive tit-bits from many people—some helpful, some useless, some dangerous—and quite a bit contradictory.

Despite this, a child's needs in the first twelve weeks are relatively simple: food, sleep, love and shelter. It is the first two of these needs which cause the most problems.

My main focus in consultations in the first few weeks of life is on the child's feeding and weight gain. In these consultations I do not talk too much about sleep. If the baby is receiving adequate nutrition and if overtiredness is avoided, then often the sleep pattern will develop to the parents' satisfaction anyway.

How the book came about

The writing began almost by accident—actually a couple of accidents—combined with a learning curve.

A number of years ago my wife and I went to New Zealand for our honeymoon. To our very great surprise, she had a positive pregnancy test two weeks after returning to Australia. Accident number one.

Events proceeded normally for us. My wife had a fairly rocky pregnancy, but at approximately the right time our son Ben was born. He was a beautiful baby and, being the doctor in the house, I began to give advice. Accident number two.

It quickly became obvious that my medical expertise, which worked satisfactorily in the hospital, the operating theatre or casualty area, was sadly lacking at home. My wife had no hesitation in smiling at me lovingly, and completely ignoring everything I said. I had entered the learning curve.

Being a father, eventually of four children, was a major joy. At the same time I had the pleasure of delivering and caring for babies in my professional life. As I learned more from my wife's wise care, from my patients, and from many hundreds of children, I gained enthusiasm for and confidence in the area of caring for the normal newborn.

The number of families who saw me for problems of infant sleeping gradually increased, until now it dominates my consulting work. As I saw more families, the age of the children who were being brought to me increased and the emphasis expanded from *preventing* sleep problems to *resolving* those which were established.

The final event leading to my beginning to write was a complaint from a patient that I had told her too much when she was so tired. She asked me to make her some notes. So I did. Later the notes grew and grew, and here they are.

Structure of the book

You are not expected to sit down and read the book from cover to cover. Instead, look at the one or two chapters which seem most appropriate to you right now. These chapters have been written to be fairly complete in their own right, even though this approach requires a certain amount of repetition.

The sequence of chapters approximately reflects the sequence in which I handle children's problems. The early chapters thus focus on feeding, nutrition and weight gain.

For this reason the chapter on starting solids comes early in the book, to keep it logically with the chapter on feeding, even though it relates to the older infant. Issues about sleep are then discussed at length later in the text, even though this may be where many of you wish to start.

Issues of sexuality and parents' needs are discussed in a chapter of their own because they are so important. A child is an extension of a family. A child will thrive only if the family is successful. It is difficult for a family to thrive if the parents are not receiving adequate rest, nutrition and emotional support. Some of the issues of loving are not obvious and I hope some of you find that section helpful.

Above all else I wish you well with your parenting. May your child or children bring you much joy. If you are having trouble at the present, this book may help return some sanity to a situation which I know can sometimes be more than you ever expected. I believe that having children is mainly for the joy of it. So let's enjoy them. If it's not fun at the present then let's see if we can't change things a little so that the joy returns.

Food, feeding and breast care

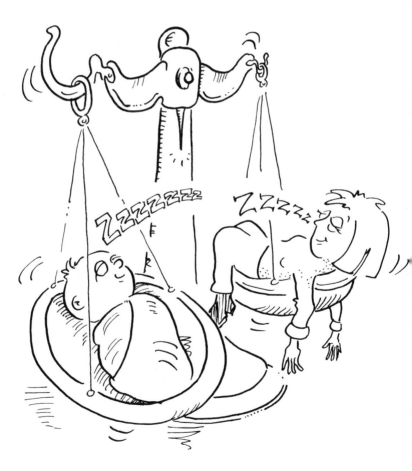

GOOD SLEEPING PATTERNS can be achieved only in the well fed baby. The first step, then, is to determine if the baby is well fed. This is where I usually begin my consultations.

A child grows rapidly in the womb before birth. The newborn will continue to grow rapidly.

The source of nutrition for this growth varies with the child's age and the mother's circumstances. There is no debate that the best source of nutrition for the newborn baby is breast milk from a healthy mother. The complexity of breast milk will never be equalled by an artificial feed. This is partly because breast milk varies according to changes in the environment of the family. For example, if the mother comes into contact with a virus she will develop antibodies and pass a degree of immunity on to her child in her milk. This is impossible with artificial feeds.

If breast milk is available then the next requirements for the baby to achieve good growth are quantity and quality.

Breast milk quantity

Most women in our society are able to eat well. Their bodies are presented with enough kilojoules and nutrients to allow the breasts to produce milk. However, each woman is unique, and the ability to produce breast milk varies. Some women are so well supplied with milk from their breasts that they could feed twins easily. Other women are unable to produce useful *volumes* of milk despite their best efforts. This variation is due to normal differences between individuals. Some of us are tall, some short, some produce large quantities of breast milk, others produce only a little.

Breast milk is the best feed as long as there is enough of it. The volume being delivered to the baby can be checked easily and in a number of different ways.

Checking quantity by observation of the baby

The volume of milk required varies with the baby's weight and the number of days after birth. A number of observations of the infant can indicate whether the milk supply is adequate.

Urine

The normal, adequately fed baby passes urine as often as every fifteen minutes. Despite the parents' best efforts, which may include nappy changes as often as 12 or more times per day, the baby is 'always wet'. This indicates that the child is probably receiving an adequate volume of milk.

Bowel action

If the bowel is being presented with adequate volumes of milk it will produce a soft, yellow, non-offensive bowel action at least once per day and often more frequently. If the bowel action is hard, small and difficult to pass, this suggests that the total volume of milk may be inadequate.

Body shape

A baby receiving enough nutrition becomes rounded and chubby. Thick cheek pads form and the arms and legs fill out.

Behaviour

The baby's behaviour is an excellent indicator of the adequacy of milk supply. If the child is well enough to suck and swallow vigorously, becomes settled and 'sedated' by the feed, settles to sleep quickly, sleeps for say 3–5 hours and then wakes to feed vigorously again, then milk supply is probably adequate.

Conversely the baby's behaviour may suggest that milk supply is inadequate. If the child is irritable at the breast, unwilling or too tired to drink, sleeps before the feed is finished or fails to settle within 15 minutes of the end of the feed, sleeps for only 1–2 hours, then milk supply may be inadequate.

The underfed baby

Underfed babies can be divided into two groups.

Underfed but coping

This baby is going to give you a hard time. He is not getting enough and plans to do something about it. The baby demands the feed vigorously, sucks hard, may continue to demand after the feed, settles poorly, and wakes early demanding the next feed. If measured, weight gain is often less than 20 gram per day.

Underfed and not coping

This situation is very dangerous. The child demands weakly or not at all. The feed is poor and is interrupted by episodes of waking the baby. The child sleeps quickly and sleeps through the next feed time. Production of urine decreases, bowel actions tend to be small, irregular and difficult to pass. If measured, weight gain is low or negative, for example less than 10 gram per day or even losing weight.

This problem needs to be recognised and treated with additional feeding.

Check on milk quantity by weighing

If in doubt about milk volume, measure it. If the volume is inadequate the mother needs to know so she can take remedial action. Conversely, the knowledge that the milk supply is excellent will cause no harm and must boost the confidence of the mother.

Baby's weight

If the baby is gaining adequate weight on a daily or weekly basis then the milk volume is adequate. I set as a base line a weight gain of at least 30 gram per day. If the average weight gain is 30 gram per day or more over several days then the mother can be reassured that her milk supply is adequate. Weight gain over 30 gram per day varies greatly, and 30, 40, 50, 60 gram per day or occasionally even more may be normal for a particular child.

If the weight is less than 30 gram per day over several days then the milk supply *may* be inadequate. A weight gain of 15 gram per day or less is almost always inadequate and requires remedial action. However, very occasionally a child from parents with small body size may be happy and thriving at a weight gain of 15 gram per day.

Test weighs

In hospital the baby can be weighed before and after a feed to give the weight of milk ingested. A series of test weighs done over 24 hours rapidly answers the question 'Do I have enough milk?'

Breast milk quality

Milk quality relates to energy density, or the ability of milk to deliver kilojoules to the baby.

Occasionally the breasts will produce an adequate volume of milk but it is of poor energy density. This tends to be determined by genetic factors and cannot be altered no matter how hard the mother tries. It is similar to height or eye colour in that it reflects the complex genetic factors she has inherited from her parents. If the genetic pattern determines that breast milk energy density is low then it can't be improved by trying hard, any more than we can change our height by working out in the gym.

Sometimes for no easily defined reason a woman will have a 'poor' lactation. With the next child the milk production may be very different. I have certainly cared for women where one lactation was difficult but another was successful.

What to do about inadequate milk supply

Imagine that we have diagnosed one way or another that the milk supply is low. What do we do about it?

It is often argued that milk supply increases to meet demand, but that is only partly true. Milk supply may be inadequate for one or more of three reasons:

- inadequate energy or fluid intake
- excess energy expenditure
- genetic factors which determine a low breast milk output.

Inadequate energy intake

It is difficult to exaggerate how busy a mother is. The amount of work increases with every child. Once a mother has two or three children, a partner, a house, a social circle and perhaps some employment responsibilities, she has become so busy that she is really being asked to do the work of more than one person. In some cultures the mother's responsibilities will be spread among other members of the group while she is given some months to concentrate on feeding and caring for her newborn. Our society does not provide that luxury.

The human body has a given number of energy units to spend each day. Some of those energy units will be used in the breast-feeding mother for milk production. Milk production will suffer if the total number of energy units available to the body is inadequate.

A breast-feeding mother should eat three meals per day.

These should contain contributions from the five basic food groups: protein, vegetables, dairy products, cereals and fat. The volume should give the mother adequate kilojoules to fill her energy needs. She should choose fluids that give energy as well as water. Milk, ice-cream, milkshakes and egg nog all provide kilojoules as well as fluid volume. I recommend at least a litre of milk-based fluid per day. If you do not like milk, then cheese, yogurt or ice-cream can act as alternatives. If you are not thirsty enough to drink a litre per day, salted nuts will help create a thirst and at the same time provide energy.

Occasionally a woman is attempting to lose weight and may be drinking only water to decrease her total kilojoule intake. In this setting the baby is feeding well, has ample urine and bowel actions, but is not settled and has poor weight gain. Dieting is rarely required in the breast-feeding mother. Her body's allocation of energy to the production of milk and the other tasks associated with a newborn infant usually means that she is often losing weight anyway. I generally ask a woman to put off dieting until the baby is gaining weight well, started on solids, and sleeping at least ten hours per night.

Excess energy expenditure

How many mothers say to each other 'What did I do with my time before I had children?'

The work of caring for children, house, partner and possibly employment uses energy. Even if her diet is providing adequate kilojoules and nutrients, a mother's milk supply can still be impaired by an excessive work load.

The single most helpful strategy when life is too busy is to sleep. For the first few weeks of her baby's life, the mother will have disturbed sleep as there are feeds every three to four hours. If at all possible, the mother should join the baby in a daytime sleep. Two hours' sleep in the early afternoon can be very humanising.

As the number of family members increases, an afternoon sleep becomes both more necessary and less possible. When an afternoon sleep is impossible, going to bed at the same time as the children can be helpful until the baby is sleeping at least eight hours at night.

Genetic factors affecting milk production

Being female, having a baby and having breasts does not mean that all women can produce milk. Humans vary in their abilities for every measurable parameter. Some are tall, others short. Some are dark, others light. The ability to produce breast milk and its energy density are biological parameters which vary from woman to woman. Therefore it is not surprising that some women produce more and others less. A 90 kg woman with pendulous breasts may have little milk supply despite her best efforts. A 60 kg woman with small breasts can often be an excellent breast feeder, to her own surprise.

Measuring the baby's weight gain and test-weighing feeds can help inform a woman of her breasts' ability to produce milk. If there is little intrinsic milk production then she should be informed so that an alternative can be used. Nothing can be more cruel than insisting that a mother attempt breast feeding when her breasts just do not produce an adequate volume of milk in any circumstances. She feels frustrated and a sense of failure; the baby fails to grow and is unsettled. The family becomes unhappy.

There is no guilt in not producing breast milk any more than there is guilt at being 150 cm or 190 cm tall or in having black hair. If low milk production is the woman's norm, in this pregnancy, then so be it. Alternatives need to be found.

This does not mean that breast feeding must fail completely; it may still be partly successful if supported. In addition, inadequate milk supply in one pregnancy does not always mean that there will be an inadequate supply in the next pregnancy.

Alternative strategies for breast feeding

Let us assume that an imaginary healthy, happy, growing baby requires 100 units of milk per day. If we measured the milk production of 100 women we would find that some could produce 200 units of milk. Some would produce very little. There would be a large majority whose production was near the 100 units required. There will be a significant minority who under ideal circumstances produce less than the 100 units which our imaginary baby needs. These women *are* producing breast milk. It is of good quality and is beneficial to the baby. However, there is not quite enough.

I have never understood why feeding should be seen as only fully breast or only fully bottle. If a woman is producing good *quality* breast milk but in slightly inadequate volumes, why not complement it with an alternative feed? There are many good milk substitutes on the market. They are not as perfect as human milk but they can be a very adequate supplement and if necessary can be the basis for total feeding. Some mothers will find that if they supplement from the bottle immediately following the breast feed the baby settles well, sleeps deeply and awakens to feed efficiently at the next meal time.

This pattern can be made a little more specific. The supply of breast milk tends to decrease in the late afternoon. While the morning feeds may be adequate for the baby's needs, by late afternoon the milk supply may be insufficient to supply the baby's whole requirement. Tea-time can become less than the ideal family event. Baby has fed but is unsatisfied and crying. The children home from school are tired, demanding and hungry. You are tired, having been up once or twice overnight. It is a fun time—the sort of time of day when being alone in the Simpson Desert seems the easy option. One step in improving this time of day can be complementary feeding at the baby's evening meal. If the baby has settled after an adequate feed it becomes easier to concentrate on the needs of the rest of the family. So the suggestion here is to give a breast feed before starting to prepare the evening meal. Follow the breast feed with a complementary bottle feed to the volume the baby desires. It might be 20 mL or it might be 100 mL. The correct volume is the one that allows the infant to settle and returns sanity to the family.

For those babies where weight gain is a little inadequate, a top-up for all p.m. feeds, that is between 12 noon and 12 midnight, can support the milk supply through that part of the day when it is at its lowest ebb. The baby receives normal breast feeds overnight and in the morning. This is the time when the mother is most rested and has the best milk supply. From 12 noon onwards, when her milk production may be starting to decrease, offer a complementary or top-up bottle after the breast feed.

Because the top-up bottle is given *after* breast feeding, the baby's demand for breast milk is not reduced. There is no need to fear that using a bottle will cause the milk supply to dry up.

Breast care

Breast feeding should be a pleasant, relaxing time. Enormous satisfaction can be gained watching and feeling a baby suckle contentedly and then sleep soundly in a relaxed pose. It is a time when love blossoms, life's worries retreat, and you just know that this is what you want to be doing at this particular time in your life. If you are tearful, upset or in pain things need to change. If your baby is unhappy, angry or unsettled, there is a problem.

Pain

Breast feeding can be sore if the nipple becomes cracked. The pain is most severe as the baby attaches to the nipple. If cracked nipples are left untreated feeding can become impossible. Nipple care is best carried out before the problem develops. In those years that I provided hospital care, the time that a baby was allowed to suck increased from a starting point of about three minutes per side on the first day. This increased by about 2 minutes per side per day until the feeds were approximately 10 by 10. This allows the skin of the nipples time to adjust to the new requirements being placed upon them.

Anyone who has suffered from dry cracked lips as a consequence of excessive licking knows that sucking removes moisturising oils from the skin. Skin that is no longer oily becomes brittle and prone to cracking. The loss of oil from the skin allows more water to evaporate and the skin dries out.

The skin covering the nipple is thinner than skin in most parts of the body. Because it is so thin it is very prone to water loss and then cracking. Such painful cracking can be avoided by applying an oily substance to the nipple. Many agents such as wool fat, lanolin and moisturiser are used in different institutions for keeping the skin of the nipples moist and oily. Even breast milk massaged into the nipple may be useful. I have had the best success with a proprietary product containing a local anaesthetic and an anti-inflammatory in an ointment base. For more specific advice please see your health care provider.

Frustration

Mother

If you are frustrated by breast feeding perhaps you should review why you are doing it. Occasionally a woman finds breast feeding unattractive and unpleasant. A sense of obligation is not the best motivation for breast feeding. More commonly a mother who wishes to breast feed feels frustrated because it is not working for the baby.

Baby

Very, very few babies will fail to display a sucking reflex. Even the most immature babies born before the reflex develops will begin to suck at the appropriate time. This reflex will be reinforced by the satisfaction of swallowing milk, making the behaviour pattern stronger.

It is not uncommon to see a mother whose baby is getting angry at the breasts. Mother is upset because, despite her best efforts, feeding times have become a time of dispute between her and the baby. The common scene is that the baby comes to the breast hungry. Initially there is strong sucking, but after one or two minutes the baby comes off the nipple and starts to cry. After some persuasion she re-attaches, but after a short time comes off and cries vigorously. Further attempts at re-attaching are not very successful and the baby turns away from the nipple. If the other breast is offered, after a short interval the same performance is repeated. The mother can often see milk on the nipples and in the baby's mouth and believes the supply is adequate.

The most common causes in this setting are inadequate milk volume, a slow let-down of milk, or an overtired baby. Another problem which can exist is flat nipples. These can make it very difficult for the baby to attach and medical assistance may be required. The diagnosis and treatment of inadequate milk volume and overtiredness are dealt with specifically in other parts of this book. The easiest diagnostic step is to offer a bottle. If the baby feeds well from the bottle, then the problem is probably a milk supply that is slightly less than the baby needs.

Starting solids

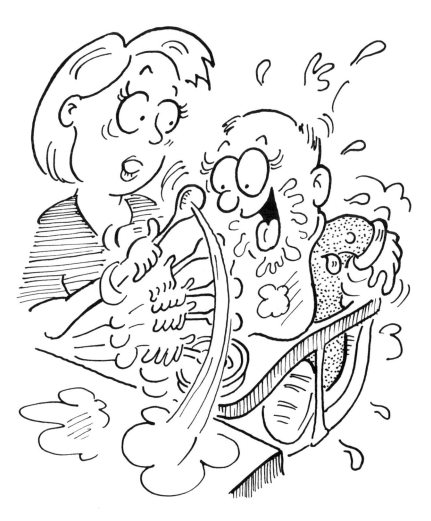

FOR SOME CHILDREN the time to commence feeding with solid food will occur sooner and for others it will occur later. When I was a medical student, one of my lecturers made the point that if the child has teeth, nature is probably giving you a strong hint. There is no set and rigid time that a child should or should not be consuming solid food, but the last section of this chapter gives some guidelines.

I try to encourage children to be sleeping between 10 and 12 hours as an unbroken block of sleep at night by three months of age. (This may include one 'roll-over' feed.) The majority of children can achieve this target, with guidance. Some children may start on solids early in their lives as a part of achieving this sleep target. This will depend on the amount of breast milk the mother is able to produce and the amount of growth that the child's genetics are attempting to achieve.

Assume that the child has achieved 10 to 12 hours sleep at night and is fully milk fed. At what stage do we start solids for this child? The answer is that we allow the child to determine the age for progressing to this next stage of feeding. We wait for a cue from the child that he is not receiving enough total nutrition. The cue which we will use is a change in the child's night sleep pattern. Whereas he has been sleeping for the whole night for many days or weeks, for no apparent reason there is a change. He is well, has had good days, and we know or believe that he is not overtired. He begins to wake during the night. Despite being in a good sleep pattern at night for some time, he is seriously awake in the middle of the night and is very difficult to settle without a feed. Instead of 'crying down' from the episode of wakefulness he 'cries up', becoming louder and more demanding. You may recognise a 'hungry' cry. The answer to this problem is definitely not to re-start night-time feeds on a regular basis. You may feed once or twice at night to convince yourself that hunger is the problem, but then you need to switch the focus to the starting of solid foods during the day.

Feeding volume

For a couple of reasons a child starting on solids will initially need only a small volume.

First, the child needs only a small addition to the breast or bottled milk that the mother is providing. Second, the child's digestive system does not contain adequate amounts of the chemicals needed to break down the new foods so that they can be absorbed. The bowel is able to produce the chemicals, called enzymes, if it is given a gentle hint that a new food is to be introduced. A small volume of the new food can be given at any one time. Over a number of days the gut will develop the digestive enzymes required for that food and the child will be able to handle a bigger volume. Sudden changes in the type of food that a child receives or increases in the volume given could be counter-productive. There is no point in being over enthusiastic and making her sick. You will lose confidence and then there will be a delay in progressing to the next stage in her development.

Consider this example from adult life. Imagine that you have not eaten meat for a long time, say for some months. Suddenly you eat a big volume of fatty meat. This can be a very nauseating experience. Part of the reason is that the body is producing less of the enzymes required to digest the meat and fat.

The initial volumes of solid food are quite small. On the first occasion the child may only consume one half teaspoon of food. Do not expect her to cope with a new feeding implement and a new food taste on the first occasion with speed and enthusiasm. She will probably cross her eyes, make a funny face and 'tongue' the food forward onto the teaspoon from which it came. This may be accompanied by an expression of surprise. Occasionally a child will take to solids at the first time. Often, however, the baby's face gives a wonderful display of emotion as she tastes a new flavour and texture. It may take two or even three days before the penny drops and her expression becomes one of enthusiasm. She will then move the food to the back of the mouth and swallow with greater efficiency.

The child is now able to commence solids regularly. The volume which you give will depend upon the baby's interest and the routine you establish. Increase the volume at a slow regular rate. At the end of the first week the baby may be taking only one teaspoon and continue to increase at that rate. Routine is useful because babies function best with a sensible, predictable routine. For example, once the solids have started, let them be continued. Do not give solids for a couple of days and then miss for a few days. Do not give the solids only on those days when the baby 'looks' as if she needs it.

Timing

Pre or post breast feeding?

When to give the solids while still breast or bottle feeding is a complex question.

Initially the solid feeding is an *addition* to milk feeding. The breast feed is given first and the solids are a top-up. At this stage most of the child's energy requirements come from milk.

At some stage the combination of solids and fluids other than breast milk need to become a more important source of kilojoules. A time will be reached when solids are given first and breast feeding is given second. The timing of this changeover is not critical, but tends to be approximately six months. Some mothers give solids before the breast feeding from the very beginning and claim that it can be very successful and does not interfere with their breast feeding.

Morning, noon or night?

One of the major reasons for deciding to start solids is to assist in the achievement of a full night's sleep for the child and thus the parents. As a parent I thought a full night's sleep was a great idea. Don't apologise to anyone for seeking a full night's sleep. If the parents are fresh and in good humour they are far more likely to provide good parenting.

I believe that it is logical to give solids at the evening meal. The child thus has a supply of nutrition in his stomach to settle for the night. Yet again this issue is not critical. Some mothers give the solids in the morning and argue that it is just as successful.

Taste

The taste of the baby's food can be a factor in determining your success. If you have tasted human breast milk, you will have noticed a significant and pleasant sweetness. The taste is about half-way between cow's milk and cordial. I generally recommend that parents place a couple of drops of milk onto a fingertip to taste. It can be helpful to mimic this degree of sweetness in designing the baby's solid foods. For vegetables, if a potato is being used as the base, then some apple, pumpkin, or carrot can be added for sweetness. If using rice cereal, which by itself is bland, a little apple puree or banana pulp may give it a little more interest. Introduce one vegetable at a time to detect any intolerance. I tend to avoid adding sugar to sweeten foods.

Consistency

Infants are not keen on lumps. Most babies will be on at least some solids before they have teeth. The food should be a fine puree, particularly when first started. This can be achieved using a food processor, vitamiser, or forcing through a sieve. In addition to avoiding lumps, the child requires a mixture which is reasonably fluid. For first solids I generally recommend a consistency similar to thickened cream.

Food choices

What solid food to give young children is an area of great discussion. Foods which are commonly used in our society include rice cereal, various fruits and vegetables, and some other cereal foods. Common sense must prevail and many adult foods are not considered. Young infants certainly have less ability than adults to handle salt and what some physicians refer to as a solute load. What this means is you should never add salt and you should choose foods with a high water content. For example, vegetables are often 80–90 per cent water by weight.

There are many fine books on infant feeding which I will not try to equal. The most specific I will be is to describe what we used for our own children. Even though my wife had a very generous milk supply, we started solids early as part of encouraging night sleep. We used vegetables to start. Boiled potato was vitamised with some other vegetable such as pumpkin, or maybe apple. One advantage of mixed vegetables is that they can be frozen as ice cubes and in an emergency 'tea' can be produced from the freezer in a couple of minutes by using the microwave. After vegetables we used Weet-bix (as a whole-grain unsweetened cereal) made into a creamy paste with milk. This tended to be the breakfast meal, vegetables at the evening.

There are many variations on this theme.

Foods to avoid

Babies have a limited ability to handle salt. Do not add salt to infant food. For the majority of infants there is no need to add butter or margarine. Avoid foods which may have a strong flavour. Baby food tends to be fairly bland. Meats, fats and most adult food will be introduced slowly, well after six months.

Food volumes

Once the baby is started on solids the volume will increase slowly but steadily. Remember that growth is hugely energy expensive. It takes a lot of food to build a body, even a small body.

Do not be surprised if the baby, once started on the solids, comes to believe that they are a really good idea. The volumes which are taken are sometimes large. It is not uncommon for a healthy baby of six to nine months to be taking almost as large a volume of food as an adult woman, in addition to breast or bottle milk.

With volume goes speed. Once solids are a regular part of their nutrition, many babies want them delivered fast. The spoon can become a bit of a conveyor belt. If you are too slow you will hear all about it. I am told that feeding twins can be fun, where it is almost impossible to keep up with the needs of two mouths.

Beware of increasing volumes too quickly. Some babies will believe that the food is a good idea and eat greedily to the point of being sick. That is counterproductive. You set the upper limit. If the baby is finishing all that you offer, add a little more each day so that the volume gradually increases. For the majority of feeds the baby will lose interest at the appropriate point and simply stop opening her mouth in response to the spoon.

Once solid foods are a regular feature on the menu, you will also set the minimum volume. On some days the baby will not be so interested. Do not be discouraged and gently persist. Try to achieve at least half of her normal volumes.

When to start solid foods

I have left this to last because it is controversial. All that I can say is that my private, unpublished research shows that the majority of babies are receiving solid food by four months. These results come from a survey of over two hundred city and country families which showed the following:

- 14 per cent of babies had started solids at two months or younger.
- 47 per cent of babies had started solids by three months.

- 73 per cent of babies had started solids by four months of age.

The specific answer depends upon a number of factors. The most important variable is the baby's weight gain. If the child's weight gain is low then start solids a little earlier.

If the weight gain is excellent and the sleep pattern is evolving nicely, delay solids. These babies are fairly easy in that they make the decision themselves. Their sleep gradually develops. Let's say they are being perfect, with eight hours straight sleep at eight weeks, ten hours at ten weeks, and twelve hours at twelve weeks. Then out of the blue they begin to wake up at, say, 2 a.m., genuinely hungry. This is the signal. Time to start solids please, Mum.

This gives us three groups of babies.

- Solids started a little early, say eight to twelve weeks of age, to supplement breast milk if weight gain is poor.
- Solids started a little early, say eight to twelve weeks, to encourage longer night sleeps. These children will often be gaining weight well, but are still unsettled. Given more food they gain weight at an even greater rate, and become more content and sleep longer.
- Solids started late, from twelve weeks to six months. These babies did perfectly and then began to wake hungry through the night.

Sleep basics

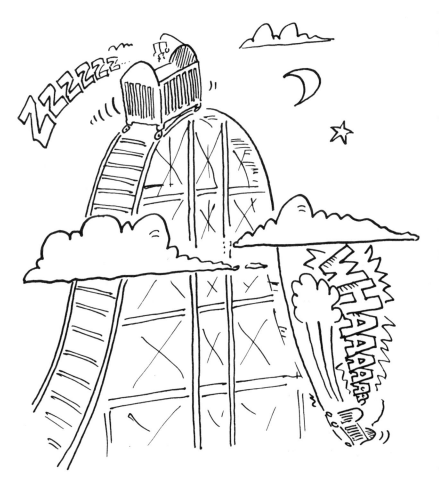

GOOD QUALITY SLEEP is necessary for the baby's growth and development. I do not believe that it is necessary to tell any new mother reading this that sleep is essential for well-being.

An understanding of sleep will help you gain control of your child's sleeping pattern. Understanding why you are helping your baby to learn the skills of sleep will greatly increase your chances of success.

Sleeping

What happens when we are asleep?

Sleep is a complex process that has different parts to it. Doctors sometimes divide sleep into levels such as REM or NREM, for Rapid Eye Movement or Non Rapid Eye Movement. Another way of defining sleep components is simply 0, 1, 2, 3, or 4, where 0 is awake, 1 is sleepy, and 2, 3, or 4 are different types of brainwave pattern or activity during sleep.

In this chapter I will focus on what I regard as some essential characteristics of sleep. These can be summarised as follows.

- A normal block of sleep contains multiple times of being awake.
- Going to sleep is partly dependent upon events around us.
- Achieving sleep is *usefully* regarded as a *learned skill*.
- Tiredness interferes with the performance of all learned skills, *including achieving sleep*.

We will return to these ideas.

Sleep deprivation

It is easiest to discuss the purpose of sleep by looking at the effects of not getting enough.

Sleep deprivation is a terrible thing. Its main effect is upon the brain, and it shows up most clearly as irritability and a decreased ability to perform learned skills. When the mind does not receive enough sleep, functioning is decreased and mood is impaired.

All of us have experienced sleep deprivation to some extent. I find that women with young children have a better understanding of sleep deprivation than men. This is simply because, on average, women spend more time attending to children through the night than do their partners. As a consequence, many women spend significant lengths of time feeling very tired while their children are young.

When we do not get enough sleep our bodies continue to function. Our hearts beat and pump blood, our lungs continue to expand and give us oxygen. The bowel still digests and the other organs of the body continue to work. The brain, however, complains. Of course there is a degree of resilience. We can all function well after losing one or two hours' sleep. However, as the number of hours of sleep loss expands and particularly if we are not able to get a full night's sleep to recover, the consequences of missing sleep increase. We all know about the tired mind. Memory is impaired. Things which we know that we know are more difficult to recall. I well recall a new mother having a difficult time who said to me, 'Doctor, I couldn't remember my own telephone number.' We all know about this as it is almost universally part of human experience to lose sleep at certain times in our lives. Most of us dislike it, although teenagers seem to need a phase in their lives where they actively seek out sleep deprivation.

It is difficult to feel positive about the world when we are overtired. The children's arguing is more difficult to handle. The pile of ironing looks even higher than normal.

Frustrations are worse than normal. Problems at home or work are more likely to reduce us to tears. Libido is decreased. Who feels like making love when we are so tired? This part of the brain seems to switch off early and turn back on late. It can be a cause of great worry in a relationship and requires great understanding and sympathy from the male partner. (This is discussed at greater length in Chapter 14, Sex and Parenthood.) I enjoyed the comment from one of my more cheerful patients and a friend who suggested that the advice to men on sex should be repeated as every second chapter to get it through to them.

Consider the effects of sleep deprivation on children. Newborn infants have very little stamina. This 'weakness' applies to all of their abilities. Would we expect a newborn child to go without feeding for 12 hours? As adults we do routinely. Would we expect a newborn child to walk 50 metres? As adults we do routinely. Would we expect a newborn to eat with a spoon without help? Babies are fragile in many ways. In particular, babies are less tolerant of sleep loss than are adults. Their minds do not have the stamina to cope well with sleep deprivation. Their mood will be irritable and tearful. Their ability to learn new skills and perform them will be decreased. Importantly, achieving sleep is a learned skill and so it, too, is affected by sleep deprivation.

Blocks of sleep

The average adult will have between six and nine hours sleep per day taken as a single block. During sleep the brain is doing many things, but we are largely unconscious of its functioning. Sleep contains periods of physical movement, periods of lying quite still, periods of dreaming, and periods of no dreaming. Sleep appears to be a time when learning is consolidated. Recent reports from the Institute of Technology in Arizona and the Weizmann Institute in Israel have shown that new skills are 'replayed' by the brain during sleep. If sleep is disrupted the learning of new skills can be disrupted.

Babies function differently from adults in many areas. Blocks of sleep are shorter. For the newborn, sleep is interrupted for feeding, which will occur at intervals of three to four hours. This is not surprising when we consider that before birth the baby received continuous nutrition from the placenta. It takes time for children to develop the reserves to cope with longer periods of fasting.

We understand as adults, particularly after parenthood, that broken sleep is not as refreshing as continuous sleep. For babies as well it is easy to observe that if their blocks of sleep are broken, then there are negative consequences. If instead of five or six *blocks* lasting three to four hours a newborn baby gets, say, ten sleeps each lasting one hour, then there are problems. These babies become overtired, are tearful, feed erratically, occupy much of their parents' time, and in particular are *difficult to settle to sleep*.

One of our aims as parents needs to be the achievement of effective blocks of sleep. These blocks need to be of appropriate lengths for both our children and ourselves. The early establishment of good sleep patterns in newborn infants is the road to sanity and happiness. Constant interruptions to sleep for our babies and ourselves lead us in a different direction.

Waking episodes

All humans from very early in life have episodes of wakefulness during blocks of sleep. This includes babies. They are a normal event in normal sleep. Understanding this will help you plan your baby's sleep pattern.

Below is a simplified graph of sleep levels for a single block of sleep. It is easiest to understand if we consider it for ourselves as adults, so think of the graph as showing a full night's sleep from, say, 10 p.m. to 7 a.m.

At the left of the graph is shown the change from being awake (0) moving through drowsiness (1) to various levels of sleep (2, 3, 4). Once asleep, our brain does what it wishes or needs. To the best of my knowledge we have no control over the activities of our brain once asleep. At some time during the night the line moves back to wakefulness (0 and 1). This waking is repeated a couple of hours later.

All humans experience waking episodes in blocks of sleep. They are short and should be silent. As adults we often forget any episode of wakefulness until specifically asked, and then

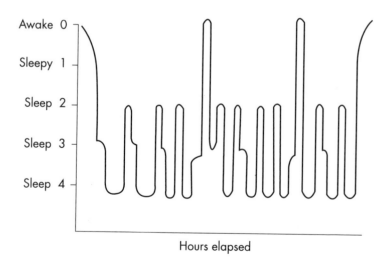

Hours elapsed

recall it is simply as a period of becoming comfortable, rolling over, adjusting our pillow or cuddling into our partner. A waking episode in a block of sleep is normally a period of hazy consciousness. We do not wake completely. It is generally a time of minimal body movement and no language. For newborn infants studied in sleep centres, there are generally two or three periods of wakefulness per block of sleep, each lasting one to two minutes. For our babies, these periods of wakefulness should be silent. You should be unaware of the child waking unless you are at the cot side.

Being awake *always* needs to be followed by a sleep transition. This means that once awake our minds go through the process of falling asleep again. For a baby a normal block of sleep will contain two or three periods of wakefulness and therefore about three sleep transitions, if we count the first sleep transition at the start of the block of sleep.

Sleep achievement

Blocks of sleep can be conveniently divided into sleep cycles. Each cycle starts and finishes with an episode of waking.

Going to sleep is a more sophisticated thing than you might think. When I ask patients why we go to sleep, they generally say because we are tired. For many mothers it is exhaustion rather than tiredness. While it is true that we sleep because we are tired, it is only part of the story.

Achieving sleep is something which we can do in one of two ways. First, there is normal sleep achievement. We feel tired, it is the correct time of day, we move to our normal place of sleeping, lie down, close our eyes, and go to sleep. For a baby this is equivalent to having a good feed and a nappy change and then being placed in the cot or bassinet.

The baby is awake and may whimper for a short time, but then goes to sleep.

The second method of achieving sleep is the sleep of exhaustion. We are tired or overtired. It is difficult to stay awake. When sitting we doze off, when we are horizontal the mind is unable to stay conscious. If we are awake we know that our mind is having trouble functioning. For babies this is equivalent to a situation which you may have seen in older children. They, the children, have been busy, active, noisy. They are walking or running around. It is late at night. When encouraged to go to bed they refuse. If put down they complain vigorously. Eventually, at 10 or 11 p.m. or later, they crash. The unconscious children are found around the house in strange postures. They are then carried off to bed.

For newborn babies this style of sleep occurs upon a background of sleep problems. They have short sleeps. Often they achieve sleep only with parental reassurance. The child may doze in his mother's arms or be patted or rocked off to sleep and then wake tearfully a short time later, calling the parents back into service.

There are some major differences between these two methods of sleep achievement.

In the first or 'normal' sleep transition, a sequence of events is gone through. There are a number of factors which need to be present in addition to tiredness which I will discuss under the heading of *cues of sleep achievement*. A normal sleep transition is usefully regarded as a *skill* which we learn. It contains a *learned* element. It can be likened to gently applying the brakes of a car at the correct time until it comes to a stop.

In the sleep of exhaustion the mind is grinding to a halt. It is so fatigued that it is refusing to move any further. This form of sleep transition lacks a learned element and lacks predictability. It can be likened to a car stopping because it has run out of fuel. This will always occur eventually if we don't fill the tank. It may not occur at the most convenient place and it certainly interferes with the appropriate continuation of the journey.

Achieving sleep involves a transition from consciousness to unconsciousness. For the child to develop good sleep patterns this should occur predictably, at certain times and in certain places. It is useful to regard achieving sleep through a sleep transition as a *learned* process. The sleep of exhaustion lacks the elements of a learned skill and does not reinforce the development of that skill.

Cues of sleep achievement

As blocks of normal sleep contain times of wakefulness, returning to sleep requires a sleep transition.

Learning to go to sleep sounds a strange concept. We go to sleep every day. However, I ask you now to regard achieving sleep as being dependent upon two factors. The first is tiredness. The second is everything else which is happening around you.

Tiredness does not require explanation. For many of you, as parents of young children, tiredness is a part of most of your days. It is a constant companion whom you would love to leave behind. Tiredness is relieved by sleep. This is known and understood by us all.

The really interesting part is the second factor or group of factors. The things which are happening around you at the time of sleep achievement are the *cues of sleep*.

The cues of sleep achievement for a baby may include the following factors.

- the time (e.g. following a breast feed)
- the place (e.g. in the baby's usual cot or crib)
- smells (e.g. the smells of mother and feeding)
- sounds (e.g. the normal sounds of the home)
- internal comfort (e.g. a full stomach)
- external comfort (e.g. warm clothes, tight wrappings)
- comfort objects (e.g. a soft toy or a dummy)
- parental care (e.g. holding, patting or rocking).

Any and all of these can be learned as part of the process of sleep achievement. This is the key to it all working for you, your child and your family.

Let me give some examples.

Consider yourself as an adult. Imagine that you are going to a motel or an interstate hotel. You are alone, the bed is too small, the pillow too thick, and the building next door is a bus depot. Will you achieve sleep normally? Will you stay asleep normally? The answer is no. We know from life experience that when we change the cues of sleep achievement so greatly, it is difficult to achieve sleep and stay asleep.

Now some of you may well say that the example is too severe. The situation has been changed too greatly from normal. So let's think of a less severe example.

You wake at 2 a.m. It is a normal episode of wakefulness in a block of sleep and should last between one and two minutes or even less. Tonight your pillow is gone. You reach out for it, half asleep. (You are not allowed to steal your partner's.) It is not in reach. You wake up more fully and reach for it again. Still not there. Eventually you are sitting on the edge of your bed with the light on, looking for the pillow. You find it, lie down, and quickly go to sleep.

The points I am making in this example are twofold.

The first point is that even small objects can be important parts of the process of sleep achievement. The presence or absence of a pillow can reinforce or interfere with the process of going to sleep. A pillow is one important cue of sleep achievement. In the absence of the normal cues of sleep there is *an elevated level of consciousness*. As we fail in returning to sleep we become even more wakeful.

The second point is that the elevated level of awakening is followed by *cue-seeking behaviour*. We do something to regain the cue. In this example we seek out our pillow before returning to sleep.

Now I have convinced you that cues of sleep achievement exist, my next task is to show that cues of sleep achievement are learned. Again, let's use adult examples.

Remember yourself as a single person. You sleep alone. You are used to sleeping in your bed, your room, your house. Then overnight everything changes. You are in a different bed, in a new room in a new house, and there is another body in the bed. Going to sleep is different. For some days the process of sleep achievement is interfered with (not just by your partner). After a number of days or perhaps a couple of weeks, you adjust to the new cues. You have erased the old cues and *learned* new ones. A similar thing happens when we move homes. After a few days in the new home we adjust to the different noises during the night and our sleep performance returns to normal. We *learn* the new cues of sleep.

We can see then that the process of sleep achievement is in part cue dependent, and that cues are learned and can be changed and re-learned.

What does this all mean? What is the significance of these arguments?

Let me use the following graph to develop the argument.

This graph is the same as the one on page 36 with one addition. For each of the sleep transitions or waking episodes, I have added a circle. Within this circle there are

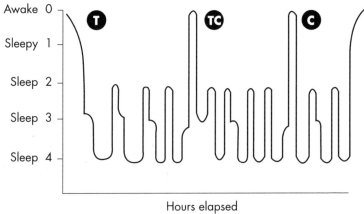

Hours elapsed

T = Tiredness   C = Cues of sleep achievement

the two influences leading towards sleep: T for tiredness and C for cues of sleep achievement. Notice the different contribution of each of these influences as the block of sleep proceeds. As adults, all of us can relate to the analysis that sleep achievement, at the start of the night, say at 10 p.m., is driven largely by tiredness. As the night proceeds the situation changes as we accumulate sleep and become less tired. Many of us can wake at, say, 5 a.m. for a minute and then return to sleep. Obviously by 5 a.m. our tiredness is largely gone. If need be, we could get up and go about our day's work. However, we don't. Children permitting, we go back to sleep. This return to sleep is partly a response to tiredness, but is now largely cue dependent.

Thus as we go further into a block of sleep, sleep transitions become more cue dependent. The cues which have been learned to help achieve sleep at the start of the block of sleep will become more significant as we move further into the block of sleep.

Let me show how this affects our care of children.

Babies rapidly learn cues of sleep in their first weeks of life. Within the first month to six weeks, styles of sleep are emerging. We can divide the cues of sleep for babies into two simple groups. The first group is those involving parental participation. Anything will do: feeding, holding, walking, patting, rocking. For the really desperate there is driving around the block. They all work. They will all provide an environment within which sleep is achieved. Parental care will be accepted by the child and learned as part of the complex process of going to sleep.

The second group of cues excludes parents. Once she has a full stomach, a clean dry nappy, appropriate wrapping, her cot, her room, normal smells and background noises, the child will achieve sleep. If these details of the environment are provided consistently *they will be learned as the cues of sleep.*

Let's try putting this all together. Our baby is normal. During sleep she will have episodes of waking which should last from one to two minutes. The transition back to sleep is partly dependent on cues from the environment around the child. These cues can be changed and re-learned. As the child moves further into a block of sleep *the cues become increasingly important* in the return to sleep from a normal arousal. If the cues of sleep achievement include parental participation then it is likely that we, the parents, will be called back later in the block of sleep to participate in another sleep transition. This clearly results in broken sleep for the parents.

The cues of sleep achievement that are most useful for baby, mother, father and family life are those that are parent independent. A baby goes to sleep with a full tummy, a clean nappy, appropriate wraps, in an appropriate bed and room, *and alone.*

Tiredness and sleep achievement

I once asked an eminent paediatric scholar about the effect of fatigue on sleep achievement in young children. He stated publicly that as they became more tired they were more likely to go to sleep. This answer staggered me. Mothers know that the reverse is true. This point appears to have received little recognition in the medical literature.

The following points are simple and useful guides in parenting.

- Children who are sleeping well go off to sleep most easily.
- Tired children are difficult to get to sleep.
- Overtired children are very difficult to get to sleep.

Now these observations are so universal in young families that I will not defend them. What I will do is try to explain why it is so.

I have argued that falling asleep is in part cue dependent and that this element of sleep achievement is learned. Now, if going to sleep is a learned skill, then it should behave like other learned skills. And it does.

Tiredness interferes with learning new skills. Overtired adults have difficulty recognising the lessons that life is presenting. This is the same for babies. As we become more tired it becomes harder for new skills to be learned.

As children become more tired they have more trouble performing their first learned skill. This is the skill of achieving sleep. The tired child has trouble achieving sleep. The very tired baby has great trouble achieving sleep. The reverse of this situation is also true. The baby who is well rested is better able to perform a learned skill. Thus the baby who is ready for bed but has not yet become overtired achieves sleep efficiently. In addition, the more often the baby achieves sleep in a given situation the sooner those cues are learned. Just as we learn our alphabet and our tables by repetition, so repeated exposure to certain cues of sleep achievement helps their being learned.

The better the child sleeps the better he sleeps. The worse the child sleeps the worse he sleeps.

I do not find many men who have experienced profound fatigue. Unfortunately a reasonable number of the mothers whom I see have experienced it. In this situation you are so tired, so desperately tired, that once you get to bed and close your eyes, you can't sleep. The eyes are closed but the mind is spinning. You know that sleep is essential, you crave it. You get to bed at last and the brain has trouble performing the skill of sleep achievement. Eventually sleep is achieved, but after much longer than normal. This is just the same for young babies. Once they are profoundly overtired they have very great trouble going to sleep.

This is why avoiding overtiredness assists in the performance of sleep skills.

Depth of sleep

Once children are asleep they become less responsive to what is happening in the house. Now just as there was a trap with tired babies being difficult to get to sleep, so the same trap exists once sleep has been achieved.

The baby who is getting enough sleep, sleeps deeply. She sleeps through telephones ringing, doors banging, TV, radio, conversations, vacuuming, and moving around in her room.

For babies who are not getting enough sleep it is the reverse. As they become more overtired they are more easily awoken. A telephone ringing, a door creaking, your footsteps—

sometimes you could swear to yourself that just the sound of your breathing—wakes them. Because they are overtired they wake easily and begin to cry at once.

It is not fair for the world to do this. Where is justice? Where is common sense? Logic suggests that the overtired baby should sleep deeply, but unfortunately the reverse is the case.

Once you understand this the solution becomes obvious. If the child is restless because of fatigue then everything else has to be put into second place to increase the hours of sleep she achieves. Once the baby has caught up on her sleep, she will achieve deeper sleep.

The child who is getting adequate sleep is easy to describe. These children tend to be calm, they go to sleep efficiently on their own, and sleep through all normal domestic noises. They return to sleep from their normal arousals in a block of sleep without help and almost always without you knowing they have been awake.

The tired baby is also easy to pick. It takes a long time for them to achieve sleep. They wake easily to normal domestic noises. They wake for their normal waking periods within a block of sleep and, being unable to achieve sleep alone, they cry.

The moral of the story is to make sure, to the best of your ability, that the baby is getting adequate sleep to perform the learned skill of sleep achievement. In the next chapter I describe sleep training and give guidelines on the amount of sleep that children usually need.

Rewarding behaviour

If you are the mother of the child it is important to understand your status. You, the mother, are wonderful. You are the most wonderful person in the world. Your smell, your touch, your milk, the sound of your voice, your warmth—to a baby these things, each and every one, are attractive, pleasant and reassuring. As a mother, and also as a father, it is a joy to feel our child's security in our arms. This is how life is. These contacts provide some of life's great pleasures and contentments.

Contact with mother or father is a reward for the child. Now, there is a time and a place for rewards. Midnight, 2 a.m., 4 a.m. and 5 a.m. are not the times for these rewards. These are times when as soon as possible after our child's birth we want and need to be asleep.

From the baby's point of view any behaviour pattern which is rewarded by parental contact is worth the effort. So if crying or kicking does the trick, so be it.

Any contact with you is a reward for your child, even if it does not include a feed. It is to your advantage not to reward behaviour that you do not want to see reproduced. If you are happy that the baby is well fed, clean and dry, is in good health and is not in an uncomfortable or dangerous position in the bed, then leave him alone. If you know that the baby is only one hour into a three hour sleep and he starts to cry a little, *do not attend* to him. Your attending to him is a reward to crying and will slowly increase the frequency with which that behaviour is exhibited. This is not being unloving but the reverse. Do you love your baby enough to allow him to learn the skill of sleep achievement alone?

The final point is more complex. If you reward behaviour occasionally, say one time in three, this is a stronger reward than if you reward the behaviour every time. Thus if a reward is given occasionally there is an increased chance of the behaviour pattern being repeated more often and for a longer period of time once the reward is finally withdrawn.

What does this mean?

If you have decided to assist your child in learning effective sleep skills and you have stopped attending to crying between feeds, then stick to your decision. If you attend one time in three or four or and give the child comfort, then the lesson that is learned by the child is 'If I cry often enough and long enough the reward will come.' The sooner the pattern of rewards is consistent, the sooner the desired sleep pattern will emerge.

Cuddles, feeding, laughing, touching, loving are wonderful. Enjoy them to the full. But they are for wake times. Sleep times are for sleep and only sleep. Love your baby enough to help him learn the skills of sleep. Babies need much more sleep than adults. They need it in blocks of at least three to four hours. By twelve weeks of age many babies can sleep ten or more hours at night in a solid block. These times are given as a guide and not as absolutes. Use them as a target to aim for as your baby and your circumstances allow.

Patient comment

'Nathan'

> I walked into Dr Symon's office a desperate and exhausted mother. To be honest, I didn't know what Dr Symon could possibly tell me that I didn't already know to help my 8 month old baby boy sleep longer at night. It was almost a relief to receive an explanation for my baby's waking and a much larger relief to find out that he would, with a little (or a lot) of persistence, learn to sleep a full night. After several weeks now of being tough and determined, our Nathan is now a much better 'night-time' sleeper. Consequently, I am a much better 'day-time' mother and wife which is very important for any family.

Sleep problems

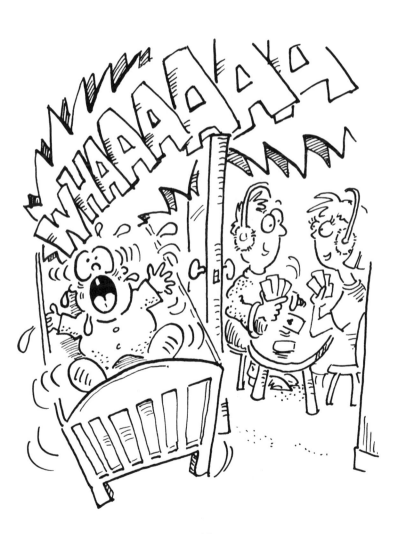

SLEEP IS ONE of life's great pleasures. Few things start a day better than waking with the realisation that you have slept well. The body feels refreshed. The mind works with clarity. Your sense of energy is renewed. Your mood tends to be more positive and cheerful—at least, until the family works you over for the two hours before they go to school.

Assuming that we get some sleep we cope fairly well with several disturbances of a night's sleep—initially. If the number of disturbances continues and our bodies or, more importantly, our minds are not allowed to recover, all of the positive outcomes of sleep move in reverse. The body is tired and listless. The mind does not work clearly or quickly and we become forgetful. Rational thought becomes more difficult. The mood becomes less than enthusiastic. Problems are approached with a negative attitude and we are more likely to burst into tears or be in a negative mood.

How many parents of young babies are left in this state? For days, weeks, months or even years?

While we can all relate to this situation, the consequences for children are less clearly understood and infrequently discussed. Some authors suggest that the need for sleep in babies varies greatly. I am not so sure that this is the case and find that the vast majority of the families that I care for find it useful to have fairly specific guides to the amount of sleep that is usual at different ages.

What is sleep for?

All of us, as adults, can relate to the negative consequences of sleep deprivation. Sleep is essential for normal brain function. I argue that it is part of the function of sleep to repair the wear and tear of the day's mental activity. There is some evidence that sleep deprivation slows and impairs brain development in some species, although for obvious reasons this research cannot be reproduced in humans. Sleep is perhaps the time when growth of brain tissue can occur most rapidly.

The newborn child is undergoing dramatic development in brain size and function. The immature, growing, brain has a greater requirement for sleep than the mature brain. In addition, the newborn has little in the way of reserves of strength to handle the unprecedented inflow of information to which the brain is abruptly submitted. Babies have a great need for sleep. Success in achieving the sleep that a baby needs is fundamental to the well-being of the newborn infant.

Mother's sleep pattern

Pre delivery

Occasionally a mother tells me that in the weeks leading up to the birth she finds that at some time of the early morning, say 1, 2 or 3 a.m., she is wide awake for no good reason. This lasts for an hour or so and then she returns to sleep. She is otherwise well and feels normal, if anyone can describe the clumsiness and indigestion of being 38 weeks pregnant as feeling normal. This change in sleep pattern may be preparation for the night feeds required by a newborn. It is not a problem and does not need treatment.

Post delivery

Almost universally the newborn will feed every three to four hours throughout the night for the first few weeks of life. The breast-feeding mother is thus woken on these occasions and misses her normal total sleep requirement. Just occasionally a baby starts sleeping through for eight or ten hours in the first weeks of life. I have received a couple of worried calls from mothers asking if it was all right to let the baby sleep. *As long as the baby is feeding well, gaining weight and normally communicative* when awake it is fine. However, for the majority, the routine of night-time feeds will go on for several weeks.

For the first baby it may be possible for mother to join in a sleep during the afternoon, thus catching up on her total hours of sleep per day. For subsequent children, when there may be a toddler or pre-schooler at home, this can be difficult. The best strategy may be to retire to bed with the other children in the early evening.

As soon as possible it is beneficial for the mother to be getting a full night's sleep. Every effort must be placed on encouraging the baby to sleep at least six to eight hours at night. For many babies this can be achieved by six weeks of age. If you expect to be feeding your baby at 3 a.m. when she is six months old, you probably will be. The importance of achieving a full night's sleep cannot be overstated. Not only does the mother feel mentally and physically better, but her milk supply improves. This improved supply then means that the baby is more rested and settled.

Baby's sleep pattern

Babies have a greater need for sleep than adults. This need is at its greatest at birth and gradually decreases as the baby grows older. Sleep requirements are at their least in adult life.

The tired adult behaves very differently from the overtired baby. As an adult, the more tired we become, the more we desire sleep. This can develop to the stage that if we sit down when desperately tired, there is a danger of going to sleep in that position. How many mothers caring for a young family and a newborn infant find that the horizontal position means instant sleep? How many fathers of young children observe that their partner's horizontal position means sleep and *only* sleep?

The overtired baby does not work that way. This is a common cause of problems in the first twelve weeks of life. The problem and the contradiction is that the overtired baby *can't and won't* go to sleep. He cries vigorously and long. He keeps the whole family awake when what he and the rest of the family need is sleep.

Establishing a sleep routine

Philosophies vary as to how a child should fit into the family's pattern. At one extreme is demand feeding and sleeping, where timing is controlled entirely by the baby. At the other extreme is feeding and sleeping by the clock, irrespective of the baby's apparent needs. From my experience the most successful path is a balance between the two.

I have been lectured to by eminent professionals on the virtues of demand feeding and constant physical contact between mother and child. I have been told of idyllic African villages where babies never cry because they are demand fed and are held in their mother's arms or on her back 24 hours a day. The only problem with this philosophy is that very few of the families I see live in idyllic African villages. Our culture sets other demands upon a mother. She is responsible for at least one child, a house, shopping, cooking, partner, and often work and other commitments. Our culture does not allow the luxury of a mother sitting or lying with her newborn for

24 hours a day for three months. Any workable plan has to recognise the constraints placed upon the mother by our social norms. For most of her conscious day the mother has to put her child down to allow her to continue with other tasks.

So what advice do I give that helps establish an effective sleep pattern?

We know that the baby has a major need for sleep in the early weeks and months of life. My observations are that for the first five to six weeks of life a healthy baby feeds and sleeps and does little in the way of communicating. To establish a good foundation to allow the development of effective communication, I emphasise the need for success in achieving a good feeding and sleeping pattern during the first six weeks.

Contact between mother and child is fundamentally important. It is essential to the normal psychological health of both the developing child and the parent. For the first six weeks the baby's important contact time is during feeds. Once the feed is finished, the nappy changed and clothing arranged, the baby needs to sleep. The mother is usually happy about that. If the baby is unsettled, there may be a feeding problem or reflux or colic. These problems should be handled as indicated elsewhere in this book. But assuming that the baby is well and fully fed, she will need to sleep at this time. Usually within five to fifteen minutes of being in bed, the well fed, healthy, tired baby should be asleep.

Other members of the family can be a problem. Playful brothers and sisters, loving grandparents and doting fathers—all must be kept at arm's length once it is sleep time. If these attentive relatives wish to cuddle and stroke, kiss and play that's fine. But this contact needs to be limited to after feed time for a few minutes only, or at bath time. Over-handling at feed times is a potent cause of overtiredness in the newborn baby.

Once the baby is fed and changed it is time to sleep. Good quality sleep for *18 or more hours per day* is as essential as good nutrition for healthy development in these first few weeks.

The temptation will occur to hold children once they are asleep. Sleeping babies are easy to love. Proud partners may wish to show off their newborn to a visitor. I plead guilty to this offence before my 'education'. The golden rule is *let sleeping babies lie!* Once sleep is established, let it continue until the next feed time.

A healthy sleep will last for times varying between two and five hours in these first six weeks. Over a period of weeks a pattern needs to be established that will satisfy the baby's requirements and leave the family routine reasonably intact. It is helpful for the mother to have a plan in her own mind so that she can develop and encourage the baby towards this desired objective.

I will discuss this plan in three ways:
- time interval between feeds (what is normal)
- age of baby (what to aim for)
- time of day (what to expect).

Time interval between feeds (what is normal)

1 hour
A baby does not demand feeds one hour apart unless there is a problem. The most common problem is hunger, i.e. the previous feed lacked adequate volume. Feeding volumes must be built up.

The second most common problem is overtiredness. The combination of hunger and overtiredness is responsible for the majority of these hourly wakenings. The irritable overtired baby can be woken by a minor stimulus and will then cry vigorously. Often parents report that the child wakes regularly after one hour or thereabouts. These children are probably waking at the end of their first sleep cycle and having trouble returning to sleep independently. They are requesting some assistance from their parents in the task of returning to sleep. These babies need to increase the total number of hours sleep per day. (See 'Overtired baby', page 61.)

Other causes include reflux, colic and a host of less common problems (Chapter 13).

2 hours

With the exception of the first two feeds of the day, a healthy thriving baby will not demand feeds two-hourly. The comments for one hour apply.

As the child becomes stronger and is sleeping eight to twelve hours at night, the first feeds of the day may change. The first feed of the day, say at 6 a.m., is a full, successful feed. The baby sleeps and then, perhaps by 8 a.m., only two hours later, demands another feed. When offered, the feed is successful. This can be seen as a catch-up feed for the one missed during the extended sleep overnight.

3 and 4 hours

Most newborn babies will sleep for at least three or four hours between feeds. The sleep should be deep, peaceful and not easily disturbed. The healthy baby in a deep sleep will ignore most normal household sounds, such as the telephone ringing, the radio on, the sound of normal conversation, or the vacuum cleaner. If the baby wakes too easily and if you are tip-toeing around the house talking in muffled whispers, the baby is probably overtired.

5 *hours*

Within a few weeks, say by three or four weeks, the thriving baby will begin to have at least one five-hour sleep per day. Ideally this will be overnight, but sometimes it is in the afternoon.

6 *hours*

This tends to occur at about five to six weeks. If the six-hour sleep is occurring during daylight hours it should be discouraged—not for the baby's benefit, but the parents'. If baby is to receive five feeds in 24 hours and there is a six-hour sleep in the afternoon it will probably mean two night feeds. You do not need that. So after four to five hours gently wake the baby (break the golden rule) and give a feed. Try to move the six-hour sleep into night-time.

7 *hours*

The baby is now six to seven weeks old and growing well. He is strong enough to sleep this long. Again the long block of sleep should be at night. There is nothing to be gained by letting the baby sleep this long in the day.

A baby who is small, thin and gaining weight poorly should not sleep this long at any time. A baby who is too weak to wake for a feed needs significant help. Seek medical advice and supervision.

8 *hours*

The thriving baby should be able to achieve eight hours' sleep at night by approximately eight weeks of age. This is a landmark in the family's return to normal sleeping patterns. The parents can have close to a full eight hours' sleep and this creates an excellent platform for the next day.

A baby who is small due to poor or no weight gain, or is feeding poorly, should not sleep this long. It is a bad sign and requires medical supervision.

9–12 hours

For the thriving baby a night-time sleep of this length can be achieved before three months of age. This establishes a night-time sleep pattern for the child for the next five or six years. Once sleeping from, say, 7 p.m. to 7 a.m., the child should keep that pattern until school age. This is another landmark in that it gives mother and father time together after the children are in bed. The return to a new but manageable family life is reasonably complete.

Note that in the first six months of life there may be a breast or bottle feed at the parents' bed time. I do not count that 'roll-over' feed as a break in a long twelve-hour sleep.

The tired, thin, underweight baby should not sleep this long. The infant is short of nutrition and needs medical assistance.

Age of baby (what to aim for)

At birth

Feeds 3–4 hourly for 24 hours averaging six feeds a day.

4–6 weeks

Feeds 3–4 hourly, perhaps a single sleep lasting 5–6 hours. About five feeds a day.

6 weeks

Feeds 3–4 hourly in the daytime. A longest night sleep of 6–8 hours. Perhaps a two-hourly catch-up feed in the first part of the day. About five feeds a day.

12 weeks

Feeds 4–5 hourly in the daytime. Ten to 12 hours of sleep at night. This may include a 'roll-over' feed at the parents' bedtime and perhaps a catch-up feed in the morning. About 4–5 feeds a day. This pattern continues until solids are started.

Time of day (what to expect)

This will vary dramatically as your baby matures and strengthens.

6 a.m.

Often regarded as the start of the day. For the newborn it is another feeding time of the 3–4 hourly routine. By 6–12 weeks of age baby is sleeping longer at night and may have two quick feeds, e.g. one at 6 a.m. and one at 8 a.m.

10–12 noon

For the newborn the 3–4 hourly ritual continues. As the child matures the feeding time will move towards the family's normal lunchtime.

1–4 p.m.

The newborn is feeding 3–4 hourly. If the mother's milk supply is decreased for one reason or another it may be a time to start complementary bottle feeds after the breast feeds.

5–6 p.m.

Perhaps the most demanding time of the day for the breast-feeding mother. The milk supply is at its lowest ebb simply because she is tired. If a complementary bottle feed is needed this is the most likely time. If necessary give a top-up feed, let the baby settle, and free up your time for the rest of the family. Remember the wisdom of having meals in the freezer and re-heating in the microwave. A little technology can help a great deal to return some sanity to this time of day.

7–10 p.m.

The newborn continues to have feeds 3–4 hourly. The more mature baby may have a late 'settling' feed before sleeping eight hours. By three months baby should be sleeping through till morning and this time can be spent in the luxury of your partner's company. There may be a roll-over feed at the parents' bedtime.

11 p.m.–6 a.m.

Feeds 3–4 hourly for the newborn, but sometimes by six weeks and usually by twelve weeks these hours should be yours for sleep.

Establishing a night's sleep

A full night's sleep is a most refreshing event for the mother. She is the axis of the family and her mental and physical health is of fundamental importance to every other member of the family. Adequate nutrition and adequate rest are the principal requirements for her health.

The baby who is thriving will be able to sleep six and possibly eight hours at night by six weeks of age.

Some babies will continue to wake at 3 a.m. for the night-time feed. Of course, angelic children will be sleeping through of their own accord, but some will not. If the baby has good weight gain, is relaxed and comfortable and is otherwise well, then you can begin winding down the 3 a.m. feed. If the baby is looking only for a dummy and is sucking lazily, give her a dummy. If she is looking for some fluid and not satisfied by a dummy, give the shortest feed that will allow her to settle. Keep cuddles and changing time to a minimum and get the child back to sleep as soon as possible. Sometimes just a bottle with some boiled water will allow the baby to settle. Another strategy, if you are sure that the baby is well, gaining weight and thriving and is simply awake for some contact, is to ignore her. Often the chubby contented baby will cry for a few minutes in a half-hearted fashion and then go back to sleep without your contact or with no more attention than a nappy change.

If you have a clear desire to achieve eight hours' sleep and are willing to guide the baby in that direction, it can be achieved. If you believe that 3 a.m. feeds are normal until twelve months, then that is what you will be doing. Remember that sleep is at least as important to the baby as it is to you. You are not being unkind by insisting that the baby increase her total hours of sleep. Everyone gains. Baby wakes next morning strong and hungry and likely to feed well. You have had a good sleep and will have maximum milk supply. Nothing starts the day better than a full night's sleep, a rapid successful breast feed, and then sitting for a few minutes gazing into the relaxed, sedated face of a well fed, thriving baby. Allowing yourself a full night's sleep is a significant contribution to the health and well-being of the whole family.

The overtired baby

Few situations cause more concern and family disturbance than the overtired baby. This problem is extremely common but I am greatly surprised at how infrequently it is recognised.

There are few areas in medicine where I believe that my advice is more helpful.

As we have seen, sleep is fundamentally important to the normal functioning of the body and particularly the nervous system. Every mother who has had children recognises the significance and disruptiveness of being overtired.

Multiple nights of broken sleep result in emotional variability, irritability, decreased rational thought, a sense of tiredness, and overwhelming fatigue. This occurs in a grown woman whose strength and stamina are much greater than that of a newborn. The baby's nervous system is undergoing dramatic growth both in size and function. Every moment awake is filled with new sensory information. All the senses are bombarding the central nervous system. The brain's ability to handle and filter information is very limited. It is not in the least surprising that the newborn is very susceptible to fatigue.

From a scientific perspective we still have much to learn about sleep. What we do know from life experience and scientific study is that sleep has an essential function in maintaining smooth, purposeful, rational brain function. When fatigued, we are able to rejuvenate during our sleep. The deprivation of sleep in the strongest and best trained of adults will eventually result in unstable brain function. Memory fades. Rational thought becomes imperfect. The ability to learn decreases. Emotional responses to situations become exaggerated and unpredictable. This is in an adult where the brain has matured and stabilised.

The newborn has much less stamina. In the newborn the nervous system is undergoing dramatic growth at the same time that it is learning to filter and process the large amount of information being presented to it. The strength to handle sleep deprivation has not developed. A baby will show the effects of sleep deprivation rapidly. Chronically overtired children may show short attention spans, varying degrees of abnormal behaviour, disordered play, irregular feeding and immature personalities. Fortunately babies also seem to recuperate rapidly once normal sleep is achieved (depending on the length of deprivation).

The presentation of overtiredness

If overtiredness is so common, what are its symptoms?

Children of less than six weeks have a limited repertoire of symptoms and signs. Often a symptom, for example crying, can represent a multitude of problems. Feeding, sleeping and crying disturbances all need to be considered carefully.

Feeding disorders in the overtired baby

The overtired baby may feed satisfactorily but is often inconsistent. The child will suck for a short time and then become sleepy before the feed is finished. The mother will know that the feeding time is inadequate and attempt to wake the baby. Conversely, the baby may start to feed but quickly become irritable at the breast and refuse the nipple. The feed may become drawn out and not succeed in giving the baby the milk volume he requires.

A crucial element here is that despite hunger and tears before the feed, the baby sleeps in his mother's arms. The overall feeling at the end of the feed is that it has been unsuccessful.

Sleeping disorders of the overtired baby

The overtired baby displays a clear and consistent contradiction in her behaviour. Whereas the tired mother usually sleeps rapidly once lying down, the overtired baby does not. *The overtired baby is very difficult to get to sleep.* This behaviour is not logical, it is not how we behave as adults, *it is not expected.* This contradiction can lead to difficulty in making the diagnosis and the ultimate worsening and prolongation of the problem.

After a difficult feed the overtired baby settles in her mother's arms. When the baby is laid in her cot she rapidly begins to cry. The crying is long and distressing. If the parents are strong willed enough to leave the child unattended, she will eventually begin to settle. After a long time, say 15 minutes, the crying stops. Despite this, any disturbances in the house interrupt the baby's sleep. These may be very minor and can include a child talking, a door opening, or even the baby's own movements. If disturbed from sleep the baby begins to cry at once. She will sometimes wake suddenly and may sound distressed. Once again she is difficult to settle.

The majority of loving, attentive mothers facing this tearful distressed child give what their hearts tell them to give—attention. The child is lifted and held or rocked in a cradle or walked around the house. The most extreme example I know of was a family who found that their child settled only when driven around in the car.

Handling the overtired baby is counterproductive. It simply prolongs the time when the baby is awake and should be asleep.

Many mothers say to me that their babies are in pain. They look upset. They shed tears, become red in the face, have a worried expression, draw their legs up. 'Doctor, there is obviously something wrong.'

The clue to the problem is the child's response to comforting. When held or rocked or driven around, they settle. How many parents have spent countless hours rocking the cradle to bring peace to the household? A child who really has something wrong is not usually pacified by simple contact. A sore ear or other true pain causes discomfort to an extent that rocking the cradle does not help.

The next clue is that when the child settles for a second time as a result of this attention, she is not deeply asleep. Within minutes of putting the settled baby down or stopping the cradle, the child is crying again. The intervention has not allowed the baby to go into a deep restful sleep. Even when the baby has started to doze in her parent's arms she has not achieved deep sleep.

Crying disorders in the overtired baby

The overtired baby is perhaps best described by comparison with a well rested baby. A baby who is feeding and sleeping well is not particularly tearful. He wakes for a feed and demands strongly but then feeds well and goes to sleep with a minimum of fuss. Once asleep the child achieves an excellent depth of sleep. People talking, children playing, telephones ringing do not wake him from his sleep.

The overtired baby has an irritable nervous system. Many minor disturbances result in crying. The crying is loud and long. The baby is difficult to settle because of his deep-seated irritability. He is so irritable and unsettled that many events result in loud, distressed crying. The crying of this baby may be similar in volume and length to a fit but ravenously hungry baby demanding a feed. It is a noise which is difficult to resist.

Examination of the overtired baby

Detailed medical examination of the overtired baby finds that ears, throat, chest, abdomen are all normal. The clues lie in the general observations. If the baby is old enough to be making eye contact, in the overtired baby the eye contact is poor. When looking into the eyes of a healthy infant of more than six weeks of age, two things emerge. There will often be a smile reflex, and the contact will be 'meaningful'.

I am not sure how to describe 'meaningful eye contact', but every mother that I ask understands at once what it is. It is eye contact that includes an emotional 'connection'. The overtired baby is very difficult to get to smile. It is also difficult to achieve 'meaningful eye contact'. These babies are difficult to establish emotional rapport with.

The second general observation of overtired babies is their movements. Babies who are well rested move their arms and legs in a smooth fashion. When they are lifted or moved their muscle tone is relaxed. The movements of the overtired baby are tense rather than calm. At the most extreme the baby may lie in the cot with a slightly worried expression and a mild intermittent tremor of the hands. When lifted and moved the baby's muscle tone is not relaxed. If the arms are quickly extended and then released, they flex with a tremor and cause the baby to cry. The healthy, well rested baby tends to lie with limbs extended and relaxed muscle tone.

Diagnoses other than overtiredness

As will be obvious to all experienced mothers and fathers, the disorders of behaviour listed above can also occur in other settings. A baby may be irritable and tearful because of hunger. Feeding may be poor because of oral thrush or tonsillitis. Sleep may be disturbed because of reflux and 'indigestion'. Colic may cause pain, and show up as an unsettled tearful baby who feeds poorly. It is the combination of medical examination coupled with the parents' observations that enables the final diagnosis to be made.

A fundamental part of establishing a diagnosis is to establish that weight gain is satisfactory. The baby must be bare weighed and a weekly or daily weight gain calculated. If the weight gain is satisfactory the focus can move from consideration of a feeding problem to tackling a sleeping disturbance. If the baby is gaining more than 30 gram per day or 200 gram per week then underfeeding is probably not the cause of distress, although just occasionally a baby with normal or tall parents may need a weight gain of 45 gram or even 60 gram per day to be satisfied.

Obviously if the weight gain is less than 20 gram per day the focus moves to feeding. As always, there is an exception. Occasionally a child of smallish parents may be comfortable and relaxed with a weight gain as low as 15 gram per day. When this occurs it will probably occur in that child's brothers and sisters as well. The overall behaviour of the child must be considered.

If the medical examination is normal and the baby's weight gain is satisfactory, if the baby is not showing signs of constipation or reflux, then the most likely cause of distress is tiredness.

Treatment of the overtired baby

The overtired baby is very easy to treat. Unfortunately few treatments are so difficult to carry out. First-time parents are hesitant to carry it out.

The treatment is no treatment.

The treatment is do nothing.

The treatment is put your hands in your pockets and walk away.

But what does this mean?

I have argued that the problem is overtiredness. The treatment is aimed at increasing the number of hours sleep that the baby receives in 24 hours.

The common approach of holding or rocking or walking

fails in the long run. Although it succeeds in soothing the baby, it fails in the long run because it does not establish sleep. The baby may relax and doze in your arms or at the breast, often when she should be feeding. However, when put down to sleep she wakes almost at once. The baby does not need a snooze, she requires hours of deep, refreshing sleep.

While the healthy, well rested baby does go to sleep rapidly in almost any reasonable circumstances, some compromises must be made for the overtired baby.

Like all of us, a tired baby will find it easiest to sleep in a quiet, dark, warm place. In addition the baby will be reassured by supporting wrapping. Take care not to over-wrap in warm weather as overheating can be dangerous.

Once in this position the mother and father must leave. The baby will cry. Do nothing. Hold each other's hands, play cards, watch TV, *but do not pick up the baby*.

The baby will cry. The crying will be loud and long. It can last for a very long time. The more overtired a baby the longer she can cry, until exhaustion takes over.

Most parents find this instruction difficult to obey. On the surface it appears unkind to leave the baby crying. You will need to have faith in me for the moment. This does work, and is not unloving. In fact the reverse is the case: helping the child to 'learn' good sleep habits is one of the kindest, most loving things you will ever do for your baby.

After a short time many parents break and 'give comfort'. This can be disastrous. Even if the baby stops crying in a parent's arms, at some time she has to be put down. Let's say the parents spend 15 minutes settling the baby. Eventually the baby goes back into the cot and starts to cry again. All that has been achieved is that the baby is now a further 15 minutes or more deprived of sleep.

There has to be an emotional outlet to this hard-line

attitude. It is cruel of me to ask parents to sit for 'hours' listening to their distraught infant. The program here is to allow contact at given time intervals. Time has to be measured on a watch, not in the heart. It is amazing how long 60 seconds of loud crying can seem.

To maintain sanity and their belief in themselves, parents must be allowed to have contact with the crying baby. But when? I recommend that the parents wait for at least 10 or 15 minutes. However the time needs to be chosen by the parents. If it is emotionally impossible to wait for 10 minutes, then try five. At the end of the time that you feel is the maximum that you can wait, go to the baby. At this time spend a maximum of one or two minutes with the child. *Do not settle the baby in your arms.* Use soothing touch or words. Let your voice convey your affection, your confidence, and that you are calm. Hold in your mind an image that the child is about to return to sleep shortly. These body language messages are important in reassuring your baby. The child may still be sobbing. Reassure the baby that you are still around and then leave. Leave the room. The next non-contact time is 20 minutes, and then 25 minutes, and so on. The majority of babies achieve sleep in the 15 minute time frame. Please try to remember that the child will not be injured by crying. Nothing breaks and nothing falls off.

This program works. It may take several nights and be emotionally very draining, but it is worth the effort.

Crying down

'Crying down' is a term which I use to describe the pattern of crying when the overtired baby is going to sleep. By creating a mental picture of the noise that will be heard, the parents are assisted by knowing what to listen for.

Crying down is in essence the reverse of crying up. Crying up is the description of a child waking from a good sleep and starting to demand feeding. Crying up starts with silence. The child is asleep. He wakes. First sounds are soft, gentle, subtle. After some time, perhaps a minute or two of being ignored, the baby begins to cry. After a short time of crying the baby will be silent for some moments. If he is ignored the crying starts again, but louder. Crying gradually increases in volume and with the gaps between cries becoming shorter until the baby is emitting a continuous loud bellow that few human beings, conscious or unconscious, can ignore. It's feed time.

Crying down is the reverse of that picture. This is the noise of the overtired baby going to sleep. The child is put down after the feed. The nappy is clean and dry. You know that the baby needs sleep. Unfortunately the child is irritable and despite his need for rest he starts to emit a continuous loud bellow that is difficult to ignore. If mother and father are attempting to sleep, the crying of the tired baby makes it impossible. Unless both partners are aware of the problem at least one will be inclined to 'do something' about the baby. Herein lies the chief pitfall. Both partners need to *do nothing* and *support each other* in doing nothing. It is amazing how hard doing nothing can be. Watch the clock; after 10 minutes you are allowed to touch your child.

The loud, continuous bellow continues for a few minutes. At some stage the child will have a short break to catch breath. The silence is short-lived and crying soon recommences. The volume may be a little less. After some time a longer break occurs. The next bout of crying may be a bit softer. The next break may be a little longer. Gradually the volume decreases and the breaks between bouts of crying become longer to the point that the baby achieves sleep. This process of crying down can take 10 minutes, 15 minutes, or

30 minutes. The length of time reflects the degree of tiredness. The more overtired the baby the more difficult it is for him to get to sleep. The more overtired the baby the more important it is to let the baby cry himself off to sleep so that sleep is achieved. The sooner the baby catches up on the total number of hours of sleep required then the more rapidly he will sleep easily.

I call this technique of supporting the baby crying down to sleep a program of minimal reassurance. There are few pieces of advice I give to the families I care for that are more important. Few are as useful in improving family harmony and allowing members of the family to get on with the task of enjoying each other. The overtired child finds it difficult to relate to his parents. His behaviour is erratic and annoying. He is tearful, demanding and hard to placate. The overtired child is harder to love.

Parenthood should be emotionally rewarding. It is the emotional richness which is the major reward of parenting. There are certainly no other rewards. In every other respect parenting is give, give, give. That's fine. The emotional reward far outweighs any cost of time, effort or money. Overtiredness in a child and then in the parent interferes with the development of the calm, happy, loving relationship which enriches our lives and makes all the effort worthwhile. The self-discipline of preventing or resolving overtiredness in a baby is essential in allowing the positive aspects of parenting to flourish. Parenting is fun. Allow yourself that pleasure.

Emotional damage

The question that is asked more commonly than all others is about emotional damage.

'If I let my baby cry herself to sleep will I damage her emotionally? It certainly breaks my heart.'

This question only occurs at the first consultation and is irrelevant by the second. I will explain.

At the first visit I usually have two tired or exhausted parents, and a tired, sleepless, irritable infant. The family unit is under stress. As parents we never stop loving our children, but when we and they are overtired it can be difficult to enjoy them.

Return to the idea that tiredness interferes with normal brain function. We all know that when we are overtired, we do not function to our full potential. The memory is faulty, emotions are fragile, frustration tolerance is lower, tears are closer to the surface, and we do not feel as affectionate to anyone. (Men, turn to the chapter on sex at this point.) Conversely, as we get better sleep, all of the above problems reverse towards normal.

A child who is overtired has the same problems but because of her immaturity is even *more* prone to the effects of overtiredness.

If several members of a family are overtired, then the chance they will interact harmoniously is reduced. The joy of parenting is to share love with a child who accepts us unquestioningly. If we are too tired to function well then those relationships do not thrive.

If I modify a child's behaviour so that she sleeps more effectively, this allows the parents to sleep well. If child and parents wake refreshed, then their relationships are improved. This includes the ability to give and receive affection. A family that is sleeping well is far more likely to enjoy each other's company.

Hearing a baby cry herself to sleep can be painful. However, it often only takes three to five nights before sleep is improved for everyone. Once the child is getting the sleep she needs, she is so much happier. The parents will then know without any doubt that they have done the right thing by their baby as well as themselves.

Once you are through the storm and out the other side, you will be totally sure that you and your children are emotionally strengthened, not weakened.

One note of warning

If you are starting with an older child, say 12 months, there may be several days where you are not so sure. The child will have eventually cried himself to sleep and slept reasonably. However, during the day the child wants you around more than normal, wants to touch and be held more. What follows is the interpretation that works in this setting. For the child, the relationship with his parents is the most important thing in life. This child had been receiving a lot of parental contact overnight. That was the problem for the family. Now suddenly the contact has been withdrawn overnight. The child's emotional world is challenged. During the day he therefore wants to 'touch base' with his parents more often to check that relationship. This behaviour, which we may interpret as insecurity, lasts a few days and then it settles, for two reasons. The first reason is that the child feels emotionally strengthened because of better sleep. The second reason is that his parents' affection is not only still present but increased because of their improved sleep.

I promise you that if you and your child get improved sleep you will enjoy living with each other more.

Patient comment

Our daughter ended up going to bed at 9.30–10 p.m. with unsettled behaviour. She was then up during the night for 2–4 hours and not having an afternoon sleep. We tried a lot

of things during the night to get her to return to sleep, e.g.
videos, milk and biscuits, following each other around the
house, bed-hopping, and ended up sleeping on the couch or
floor. Being a shift worker I could tolerate a broken sleep
pattern for some time, but it did get to a stage when my
husband and I were desperate and sick of our lifestyle.

We had tried for 2 years and weren't getting any closer to
consistent sleep, instead we were getting further away. We
were pleased to get 7 hours of straight sleep for every fourth
night. We couldn't have her in our bed like 'everyone' suggested, because she saw this as party time. We tried a mattress, beside the bed, but she still had the night-time wanders.

Someone told us of Dr Symon, so we apprehensively made
an appointment. We followed his suggestions and couldn't
believe that the procedure worked. I wish there was a 'magic'
procedure for some other undesirable behaviour patterns.

We only had to shut the door for one minute once on
that first night. Since Easter our daughter sleeps through,
she has got up at approx. 4.30–5 a.m. twice, frightened as
she had been disturbed, and came into our room. When
reassured we returned her to bed and she settled well. She
now wakes from 6 a.m. onwards and comes into our bed,
but she is more settled and appreciates this special time with
us. She now has sleeps during the day as well.

The essential advice

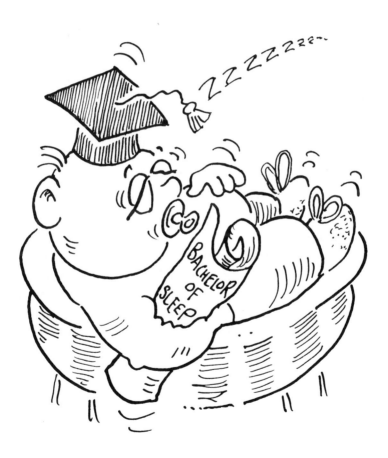

THIS CHAPTER HAS been written to present the most important elements of this book in a way that is logical and compact. While much of it has been said elsewhere in this book, presenting it in this way appears to work well for many families.

Blocks of sleep and sleep cycles

Humans require sleep, and sleep is most effective when it is achieved in blocks lasting a number of hours. Most adults, for example, feel refreshed by achieving between eight and ten hours of sleep in a single block, overnight.

In recent years, studies in sleep laboratories have found that sleep occurs at different levels during a block of sleep. In particular, all people, from birth through their whole life, experience awakenings during a block of sleep. The purpose of these shallow awakenings is not known. A block of sleep is thus divided into *multiple sleep cycles*. A sleep cycle is one circuit starting with wakefulness followed by a period of sleep and *concluding in a waking episode.*

The length of these sleep cycles varies with age. For a young baby they may be as short as 40 to 50 minutes. In adults the sleep cycles are approximately 90 minutes long. Most of us will therefore have between five and six awakenings in an eight-hour sleep, although we have little or no recall of these awakenings the next day. Despite this 'forgettability', these awakenings contain an element of awareness. It is in these episodes that we would recognise that a pillow has fallen off the bed, for example.

The importance of these awakenings or arousals with regard to infant sleep is that they conclude in a *return to sleep*. Thus a block of sleep contains not only multiple arousals but also *multiple episodes of sleep achievement.*

In a young child the length of a single block of sleep can vary from approximately three hours soon after birth to as long as twelve hours after some months. The individual sleep cycles within that block of sleep change only slowly over a period of years. Sleep cycles in the first few months of life last about 40 to 60 minutes. These cycles conclude with a shallow awakening which should last 30 to 60 seconds and be largely silent. The awakening will then be followed by a return to sleep. If the block of sleep is complete the arousal will lead to full awakening.

Cues for sleep achievement

Given that a block of sleep contains multiple episodes of achieving sleep, what helps sleep achievement to occur?

To assist in understanding and then gaining control of infant sleep I suggest two causes of sleep achievement. I do not pretend that this explanation reflects the full complexity of sleep achievement, but it leads to advice that works for most families.

In my consulting room there is normally a very tired pair of parents sitting with me. For many of the families I see, tiredness has changed to exhaustion. They rarely have any trouble volunteering that tiredness causes sleep to occur. I well recall that when our children were very young, my wife appeared to be deeply asleep *before* her head hit the pillow. None of us have any trouble agreeing with the statement that tiredness leads to sleep. Unfortunately this simple statement is incomplete and is somewhat misleading when discussing infant sleep. Despite the presence of tiredness, other things are required for sleep achievement to occur smoothly and efficiently.

Imagine you are very tired, the children are asleep, the house is quiet, all the important work is complete, and you are ready for bed and sleep. However, instead of lying down in your normal bed, in your own bedroom, for my own reasons I ask you to lie on a portable bed, in a sleeping bag, on your own, in the carport. Your tiredness is still complete, you are just as badly in need of sleep, but because the setting for your sleep achievement is so different your ability to achieve sleep is decreased.

I call the environmental factors, the setting in which you normally achieve sleep, the *cues of sleep achievement*. For normal sleep the ability to go to sleep is dependent upon a combination of tiredness and appropriate cues of sleep. The common cues are being in the right bed with normal sounds, smells, warmth, blankets, pillow, the correct company, and at the appropriate time of the day. The more we disrupt the cues of sleep the more difficult it becomes to achieve sleep. We can summarise in the following way:

SLEEP ACHIEVEMENT = TIREDNESS + CUES

Learning and changing cues of sleep

Cues of sleep achievement reflect your surroundings. Each of us has a subconscious list of cues which we recognise. These cues are learned and completely changeable. For example, as single adults we have certain sleep skills. We achieve sleep and maintain sleep in, for example, our parents' home, and we take these sleep skills for granted. At some stage we form a relationship and begin sleeping with a partner at a different home. Overnight all the cues have changed. A new bed, new bedroom, different house or flat, and two bodies in the bed. Most of us accept that our sleep skills are temporarily disrupted. It takes a little longer to achieve sleep, we are more conscious of arousals overnight, are aware of our partner turning over or snoring through the night. However, thankfully the disruption to our sleep is short lived. Within a week or two the subconscious 'reprograms' itself and our sleep skills return to normal.

I sometimes talk about an imaginary 'computer program' which has the title 'this is how I go to sleep' which we store in our brain. When we need to achieve sleep, we pull this program out from its file and use it as a reference point to assist us. When the lines in this computer program are changed, i.e. when the cues of sleep are changed, our efficiency at achieving and maintaining sleep is decreased. Then, over a period of days or a couple of weeks, we 'rewrite the program'. Old cues are erased and new cues are written in. As this new program takes shape our sleep skills come back towards normal. We do this so well that soon we *need* the new cues. For the majority of women that I see, their partners were disruptive to sleep at first, but now if he is away for the night they do not sleep as well. So in adult life, if we change cues of sleep we suffer some sleep disruption, but then relearn new cues which allow our sleep efficiency to return towards normal. Another example which most of us can relate to is the temporary sleep disruption of changing house or flat. In the new environment we rapidly rewrite our sleep program and our sleep efficiency returns to normal.

Sleep achievement as a learned skill

Sleep achievement is usefully regarded as a learned skill. This point is one of the keys in my method of caring for infant sleep. Sleep achievement is in part cue dependent; cues of sleep are learned. By combining these two points we arrive at the conclusion that sleep achievement is also learned.

Now, I cannot prove one way or another if sleep achievement is a learned skill. What is important is that if we accept this analysis of sleep then the advice it leads to works. The advice also reflects what we see with infant sleep and, to an extent, adult sleep. So for the moment let's choose to look at sleep achievement as being one of our many learned skills.

Fatigue

Fatigue interferes with sleep achievement.

It is difficult to overstate the importance of this point. This is a tripping-up point for many parents. It is a trap for the innocent and the well-intentioned. It is where the majority of infant sleep problems have their origins.

The problem is that at first glance this proposal seems wrong. Haven't we already agreed that sleep achievement is the result of a combination of tiredness plus cues?

Let us return to the idea of sleep achievement as a learned skill. If this is correct then sleep achievement should behave like other learned skills. Our life experience teaches us quite clearly that fatigue interferes with the performance of learned skills. Remembering our multiplication tables, telephone numbers, the alphabet, appointments, and what we have come to the supermarket to buy are all things we more usually associate with memory and learned skills. So let's think for a few moments about these learned skills and the effect of tiredness. Almost universally the parents I see and in particular the mothers of sleepless infants are suffering from sleep deprivation to varying degrees. Almost all of these women agree that their memory is atrocious. They are having trouble remembering telephone numbers, shopping has become a bit random and things are forgotten. They are having to write notes to themselves to avoid forgetting important events.

We know that fatigue interferes with the performance of learned skills. Now, if sleep achievement is a learned skill then fatigue should interfere with sleep achievement. Once again, this point is one we can recognise and accept from our life experience. Parents of young children are often very tired. The mothers in particular have gone past tired, have become overtired, and then exhausted. Body and soul are crying out for sleep. The following scene emerges. The children are asleep at last, the house is quiet, you badly need to sleep, you get to bed, lie down, close your eyes, and what do you find? Your mind is spinning, your emotions are confused, you are on edge, and sleep is slow to arrive. You have become so tired that it is hard to get to sleep. Sleep is eventually achieved, but it is slower than normal. During this time the mind is not relaxed and peaceful. Becoming overtired has interfered with efficient sleep achievement. Returning to the computer program called 'this is how I go to sleep', you can become so tired that it becomes difficult to retrieve that program from its file. Imagine your tired mind at 2 a.m. after a busy day asking itself 'Now where did I put that note about sleep? Just can't find the darn thing at the present.'

The relevance of this to infant care is as follows. We, as adults, can become overtired to the point that sleep achievement is difficult. Infants have much less stamina than adults, and are more prone to overtiredness. They will achieve the overtired state rapidly. For the newborn this can occur within one day or even less. The older infant and the toddler are more resistant but will eventually become overtired if they miss enough sleep.

Most parents have little trouble recognising a scene where their children have missed a sleep and are then late for bed. An afternoon birthday party is a great example. The children have been playing vigorously, much food has been eaten, they have begun to be silly, and the tears begin to flow. You know that they are tired, and then overtired, so you suggest bed. Do they go off to sleep easily? No! As their tiredness increases, their ability to go to sleep decreases. You then pay the price for the children's lack of sleep.

In terms of sleep for infants I look at three individual components:

- sleep achievement: the ability to change from the conscious to the sleep state
- sleep maintenance: the ability to return to sleep from a normal arousal within a block of sleep
- sleep depth: the ability to remain asleep despite background noise.

Being overtired interferes with all three of these elements. Thus if your baby takes a long time to achieve sleep, is tearful every 45 to 60 minutes at the end of each sleep cycle or is easily woken by normal background noises like creaking doors or floorboards, then overtiredness is often the cause.

Appropriate cues

Parent-independent cues of sleep are the most useful for family life. Children respond to cues of many sorts from an early age. By six weeks of age the hormonal cycles of the body are responding to day and night. The child has begun to return a smile, and as parents we can feel the first flickering of a personality emerging.

I divide cues of sleep for infants into only two broad groups: parent dependent, and parent independent.

Parent-dependent cues

Parent-dependent cues contain an element of protracted parental care. Common examples include patting, rocking, holding till asleep, breast feeding till asleep, pushing the pram around the house, or driving the baby around in the car. From the child's perspective these are powerful and effective cues. Children are deeply connected to their parents by emotions. The parents' attention and love are the most significant reward structures for a young child. Parental contact is more important than food and certainly more important than sleep. These parent-dependent cues are rapidly written into the 'sleep program'. The process of sleep achievement is then triggered in part by parental activity. Parental attention works. We now have a problem.

As we have seen already, a block of sleep contains multiple sleep cycles, and sleep cycles conclude in an episode of waking. The return to sleep is driven by a combination of tiredness and cues. As the block of sleep continues during the night, tiredness decreases. As the tiredness decreases, the return to sleep from a normal, healthy arousal is *increasingly cue dependent*.

If a child is using parent-dependent cues, then as the block of sleep proceeds it becomes increasingly likely that the parents will be politely requested to return to provide the care which triggers sleep. This sequence works. How many of you find that you have only to get out of bed each hour or two to pop in the dummy or pat for a few minutes to get the infant back to sleep?

Unfortunately this then fragments a block of sleep for several members of the family. You do not need me to point out that the effect on your well-being of one eight-hour sleep is different from the effect of eight one-hour sleeps.

Parent-dependent cues of sleep thus lead to disrupted blocks of sleep.

Parent-independent cues

Parent-independent cues of sleep also exist. I generally talk about these cues being a full stomach, a clean dry nappy, the baby's pyjamas, her blankets, her bassinet or cot, and her room. Say goodnight.

The child will incorporate these cues into a sleep program to develop what I call *independent sleep skills*.

During a block of sleep the child with independent sleep skills can have hourly arousals, do a cue check, find that all is normal, and then return to sleep. This process will occur silently or nearly silently. The parents can then continue with their important task of being asleep and recharging their own batteries. Given a full night's sleep, the parents feel refreshed and have more energy and affection to give. The child is thus able to receive more affection and time from a happier, stronger, more confident parent.

Parent-independent cues are thus more useful for family life.

Patient comment

'Olivia'

> Olivia has always been a relatively good sleeper during the night. Our problem was the method we used to get her to sleep! I would cradle and rock her in my arms until she fell asleep (and this would quite often take hours) and then

would very gently and quietly put her in her cot. Many times she would wake the moment I laid her down, and so then we would have to repeat the routine all over again. Our evenings were a disaster. I found myself having to devote myself entirely to Olivia from the hours of approximately 6 p.m. to 10 p.m., while my husband was left to eat dinner alone (I generally missed dinner altogether) and then clean the dishes. By the time Olivia was finally asleep, I was so exhausted that I generally went to bed as well. The evening would pass and we would be lucky if we had said two words to each other! The other reason that I was physically and emotionally exhausted was because Olivia would only allow herself to be put to sleep or be comforted by myself.

I had had enough by the time Olivia was eight months old and so decided to seek help. We saw Dr Symon and he taught us his ideas on sleep. My husband and I were so exhausted we decided to try.

Our first night was awful. Olivia cried, screamed and made herself hysterical and this just broke my heart, so I cried too. I comforted her for 2 minutes after 15 minutes of crying, left her room, and she began to cry again, however she ceased crying after about 25 minutes and was sound asleep. I was surprised, as I was expecting her to cry for a lot longer, and this was a very encouraging sign. Olivia remained asleep until morning and Mark and I were able to enjoy each other's company for the first time since Olivia was born. The days that followed were emotionally draining as Olivia continued to cry each night when I put her to bed and sometimes her cries would last for up to an hour and a half. We had our best night six days after commencing, as Olivia only cried for 10 minutes before falling asleep. The weeks that followed were wonderful because Olivia would never cry for any longer than 10 minutes when put to bed. The evenings became ours again and we were able to enjoy this time together (even though most of the time we would talk about Olivia!). I was able to enjoy some freedom and could go for coffee with friends of an evening without feeling cruel or guilty. Now that we had our evenings under control, I began working on improving Olivia's daytime sleeps by following the same procedures, and I had almost immediate success.

It is now seven months since I first began (Olivia is now 15 months old) and Olivia's sleeping habits could not be better. She used to be a child who would only sleep a half an hour during the day and now she sleeps 2 hours of a morning, 1.5–2 hours of an afternoon, and all night (from approx. 7.30 p.m. to 7–7.30 a.m.). When awake, she is an extremely happy and energetic child, an absolute pleasure to be with. This in turn makes my days enjoyable and productive and our evenings are now relaxed, quiet and simply a time we can again share together. Olivia no longer cries when put to bed, and most times she is actually eager to go to sleep. Olivia is a much happier child since we have improved her sleeping habits, and we are much happier parents. I shudder to think what our lives would have been like now, had I not asked for help when I did.

The first six weeks

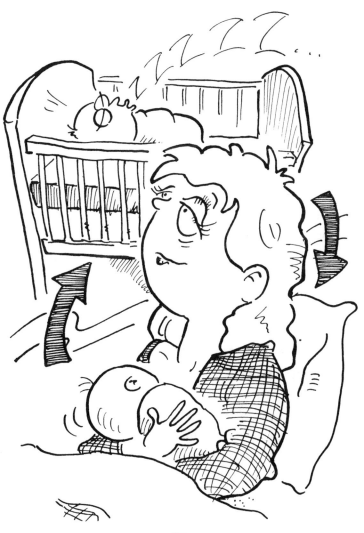

THE NEWBORN CHILD is amazingly attractive to the majority of people. Many of your friends and relatives will want to hold, touch and advise. This can be strengthening, but in excess it is tiring. As one of my patients said to me, 'every man and his dog' has an opinion about feeding and sleeping in the newborn. So do I, and here it is.

As this book is aimed at being of assistance to parents, there needs to be something to help with. If your baby feeds well, gains weight as expected, and sleeps like an angel, then there is no problem. Parents come for help when one or more of these areas is not functioning well.

Feeding is dealt with in Chapter 1, Food, Feeding and Breast Care.

The remaining problem is sleep. Poor sleep in the newborn is so common that it is almost accepted as normal. Indeed, during the first six weeks, waking for feeds every three to four hours is normal. However, long periods of crying are not expected. This first six weeks of life, in most cases when the child is normal and healthy, is a cycle of feed–sleep–feed–sleep–feed–sleep. Many families are not this fortunate and report problems with excessive crying.

I will discuss sleep problems in the newborn in two ways: prevention, and management.

Prevention of sleep problems in the newborn

Excessive crying in the newborn infant can have multiple causes. The child may be unwell. This possibility needs to be excluded. If you consider ill-health is a possible cause of your child's crying, contact your medical adviser.

Once you are convinced that the child is well but tearful,

a diagnosis of the cause is needed. Hunger and tiredness dominate. The first thing I emphasise to my patients with young babies is adequate weight gain. The prevention of overtiredness is the second thing.

Many other diagnoses may be suggested, including colic, wind, reflux, silent reflux, and minor lactose intolerance. These problems can occur, but I generally find that if hunger and overtiredness are treated, the problem of excessive crying usually disappears. In other words, I use the other diagnoses last, not first.

Hunger

The hungry infant has every right to express a negative opinion. I have already dealt extensively with this problem and its treatment. Check Chapter 1 pages 9–11 for the appropriate methods of excluding hunger as a possible cause of crying.

Fatigue

We now have a child who has been checked by an appropriate professional and deemed to be well. You have excluded hunger as the cause of distress, as the weight gain is excellent. The child is still tearful and requires much handling to settle.

The dominant cause is fatigue or overtiredness. Recognition of overtiredness is discussed extensively in Chapter 4, Sleep Problems.

Causes of overtiredness in our culture are usually easy to identify. Forgive me for stating the obvious, but overtiredness is the result of not getting enough sleep. But how do you know what is enough sleep? The majority of newborn infants will sleep between 17 and 18 hours per day, and sometimes up to 20 hours. You would be amazed at the number of raised eyebrows I get when I mention that number.

The major cause of overtiredness is overhandling. Newborn infants are a centre of attention. They bring joy, celebration, and many visits from attentive relatives. There is an unfortunate tendency for friends, relatives, partners, guests, in fact almost anyone, to want to hold the baby. Babies will often doze off in someone's arms, but they do not achieve the depth of sleep required to achieve their best rest.

Prevention of overtiredness requires some planning. It is usually the mother who has to be the policewoman, as it is usually she who copes with the consequences.

For the newborn baby, keep waking times as short as possible. Stamina is limited, and the child cannot be meaningfully awake for long at this age. Waking times in these first few weeks may be only 30 to 45 minutes. Shorter is better than longer. Waking times are for feeding, changing, bathing and enjoying touch. Once the feed is completed, the nappy changed, and the baby prepared for bed, then put him down and allow him to return to sleep as rapidly as possible. Try to avoid loving relatives playing 'pass the parcel' with your baby for hours on end. They will leave, the baby will be overtired, and then you have a difficult time because the child has become too tired to sleep well, and possibly too tired to feed efficiently.

Now some of you may be thinking or saying that your feeding takes 40 minutes. 'How can I get the child down in 30 to 40 minutes?' My experience is that the majority of babies who are breast feeding well or those who are bottle feeding will take their necessary volume in 20 to 30 minutes. There are plenty of exceptions, but the majority of babies will have taken the required volume of milk in about that time. If you find that breast feeding is taking a long time, say an hour, this is only a problem if it is a problem. If you feed for an hour and the child goes to sleep efficiently and then gives you three to four hours sleep, that's fine. Do not change anything that is working well. If, however, the baby is difficult to settle after such a long feed, there are a couple of hints.

Watch the sucking style of the infant. On first attaching, sucking and swallowing is rapid. Some of you may even hear the first mouthful 'hit the bottom' as it reaches the stomach. After several minutes the sucking will often change to a more leisurely style. The child is becoming more relaxed as the stomach fills. At some point of time the suckling becomes 'social'. To put it bluntly, the child may get to a point where you are being used as a dummy or a soother. The sucks become intermittent, and the baby is often in a shallow sleep by this time. The time taken to get to this point varies for each baby–mother team. Ask yourself whether your baby is feeding from you, or using the nipple as a dummy. If you think that the latter is the case, then draw the feed to an end and prepare your baby for bed.

Keys to preventing overtiredness in healthy newborns

- Ensure that milk intake is adequate and ensure that weight gain is good.
- Avoid prolonged handling, particularly by visitors and friends.
- Aim to achieve between 16 and 18 hours sleep for your baby per 24 hours.

Management of overtiredness

Management of overtiredness is discussed extensively in the Chapter 4, Sleep Problems, but a couple of points are worth emphasising here.

The treatment of the overtired child involves teaching independent sleep skills and increasing the number of hours of sleep per day. In the newborn, the body's reaction to light and dark is not present, but it will establish itself by about six weeks. Thus, in the first few weeks, many babies do not have a long period of sleep at night. In addition to the developing response to day and night, we now add the ability to sleep independent of the mother's body. Babies do sleep before birth, and by necessity this occurs in close and unavoidable contact with the mother. After the baby's birth I encourage mothers to allow the transition to sleep to occur alone as often as possible. If sleep is achieved in your arms, that's fine, but as soon as possible, place her down to sleep alone.

The overtired infant will have trouble achieving sleep and will protest to the best of her ability. How do you respond?

Elsewhere I have described a program of minimal reassurance, or 'crying down' (page 69). For the very young child, the guidelines are a little gentler than for the older child of say six months or more. The baby in its first few weeks is extremely sensitive to fatigue, and so prolonged periods of crying are counter-productive.

If you are happy that your baby is well, has a full stomach, and needs to sleep, then place her in her cot. Dress, wrap, and cover her in a way that is appropriate for the weather, and then leave. If the baby has gone into a deep sleep in your arms, this may be no problem at all. Sometimes, however, a baby will rapidly wake and cry. The plan of action is the same for both styles of crying. Do nothing for five minutes. If five minutes is too long for you, try three. Longer breaks tend to be more useful than shorter. If the baby has not settled in five minutes, then attend and give reassurance. Check that the baby is safe. Give a soft touch on the cheeks or forehead, let the child hear your voice. To the best of your ability, let your tone be calm, confident and loving. To a certain extent a baby mirrors your emotions, so if you are anxious your baby could become anxious; if you are calm, your baby is more likely to be calm. Avoid the traps of rocking, prolonged patting, wheeling, or walking around the house. Give reassurance and comfort for about one minute, and then leave for another five minutes. Repeat this cycle, slowly increasing the time that the baby is alone.

The majority of babies who are well and have an adequate milk supply will achieve sleep within 15 minutes, but different times of day make a difference. Settling times through the night are often shorter; mornings may be a little longer. Afternoons and early evenings may be the most difficult. As the baby becomes increasingly tired during the day, her ability to perform the transition from wakefulness to sleep decreases. Her ability to achieve sleep becomes a little weaker. This is sometimes complicated by a lower milk supply in the breast-feeding mother in the early evening. As a result the baby may be both overtired and hungry.

If you consider hunger is a potential problem, the appropriate care is discussed in Chapter 1. If tiredness is the major cause of crying, then the program of minimal reassurance as described should work for you.

After all your planning and heartache listening to the baby cry to sleep for 5 or 10 or 15 minutes, your baby will achieve better sleep skills. Once you have achieved the correct balance of milk supply, sleeping hours, and handling for you and your baby, sleep achievement will become increasingly easy.

Often families who start with this philosophy from the earliest days find that sleep achievement is not a problem, and that longer blocks of sleep, say five to eight hours long, are emerging by six weeks of age. Your friends will then reward you by saying 'But you're just lucky. You have been given a baby who is a good sleeper.'

Just smile.

Love, discipline and touching

Successful parenting is about love—by giving in large volumes and then receiving. For the majority of people, when they are counting the worth of their life it is the success or otherwise within the family that counts.

Discipline and love are interconnected. There is the self-discipline of parenting, in giving up things that were previously important for the benefit of your child, in denying your child handling time when he really needs sleep, in keeping loving relatives at arms' length when your child is sleeping. There is the discipline of establishing routine. These forms of discipline have nothing to do with punishment. Discipline as punishment has no place in the first weeks of life.

As parents, you will be presented with so much varying advice that it can be difficult to work out priorities. Elsewhere I have outlined achievements to be reached in weight gain and sleep. Often it will require significant self-discipline to achieve these aims, but the early effort is well worth it. The child who by twelve weeks of age is feeding four or five times per day, sleeping twelve hours at night and growing well has set a pattern of behaviour that may last for the next five years at least.

The whole family benefits from such a successful routine.

Our society is time-orientated. For each individual to function efficiently in a social context requires the recognition of others' routines and fitting in with them. Do not feel guilty at guiding your child to sleep and eat at particular times. By doing so the child is moving towards integration in the family unit. It is the success of the integration of individuals into a family unit which leads to the next step of moving success-fully into society as a whole. Our babies are precious individ-uals. Despite this they must fit into the routines of society at large, and their families in particular, to lead worthwhile lives.

Much is made of the importance of contact between parents and child. In some societies mother and child are in almost constant contact. I suspect that this develops a deep and meaningful relationship, but for better or worse our culture does not allow a mother the time or energy to have such prolonged contact with her baby. This is our reality. Contact time still needs to be emphasised and enjoyed when it is appropriate.

In some settings and at some times I see sleep and contact as being alternatives to each other. Many hours of good quality sleep are fundamentally important to the baby's well-being. When the baby needs sleep, allow it. Encourage the sleep to be deep, uninterrupted, and of the appropriate length. Importantly, the baby should almost always be sleeping alone.

When the baby is rested, fed and looking for communi-cation, then give as much as possible. This is the time for touching and holding. Enjoy these times. The pleasure of holding and talking to a thriving baby who is enjoying his parents' company is immense.

In the first six weeks of life, if all is going well, the baby largely sleeps and eats. At between five and six weeks most babies will begin to recognise and respond to a human face—

any human face. This is a great time. Relatives far and wide can stand before the infant, provide the smiling face and become the beneficiaries of a wonderfully cheering unhesitating smile. Everyone gives and receives undiscriminating cheer.

The party stops later in life when the child begins to recognise individuals. Thus when you are recognised as being a non-regular smiler the child will not automatically return your affection. It can be dispiriting to hear the plaintive wails of the distressed infant despite your best efforts at providing a friendly smile. It is important, though, for the child to recognise who is family and who isn't. The child cannot remain forever undiscriminating about whom he should share his affections with.

Once the smile reflex commences at about 5 to 6 weeks, meaningful eye contact develops. These are times when the baby is starting to communicate. These are pleasant contact times which are initially quite short. To a certain extent the baby will 'announce' the times when he is ready to interact. These times vary somewhat. It really can be frustrating at 2 a.m. when baby is well rested, had a good feed, and decides that it's party time. Usually, however, the happy wake times come in the day.

Recognising these times is important. Just as important is the need to recognise when they finish. The very young infant will tire rapidly. His mood can change within a couple of minutes from happy play to tearfulness. It is important to watch for this change in attitude. The baby's contact time has expired as his 'batteries have run down'. It is now time for sleep. So as rapidly as practical, change the nappy and place the child in bed.

The danger in delaying sleep is the problem of overtiredness. If the cue for bed is missed or you are simply too busy to put baby to bed, he may become overtired rapidly. Once this has occurred the child may be more difficult to get to sleep. The irony is that the child who is not overtired but who is ready for sleep and has had a good feed settles well. The overtired child may become irritable, can cry vigorously, and may be difficult to get into a deep restful sleep.

Feeding times are the other time of contact. Breast feeding is a very pleasant time when all is going well. Conversely if things are not going well it can be a time of frustration, pain and tears. For the vast majority of women, most feeds are successful and this is a time of intense closeness. The physical handling of the baby is an important step in developing bonds between mother and child. It is part of the child's learning about physical contact. Whenever possible enjoy these times to the full.

While emphasising the need for contact and its contribution to the child's and parents' well-being, it is equally important to highlight non-contact time.

If the child is due for a sleep, or is asleep, everyone should be kept at arms' length. Let the sleeping baby sleep. Repeated interruption of sleep is a potent cause of overtiredness. Playful brothers and sisters, doting partners and attentive grandparents need to be kept away. This can be difficult in the first few weeks when the baby is so new and special. It is very important that you protect the child from overhandling. This is particularly so as you have to cope with the consequences if the baby becomes overtired.

Contact time for relatives occurs at feeding times—when baby is awake and resting between sides or after finishing the feed, while you are organising the cot, or the baby is simply happily awake. As the baby grows and becomes more resilient so there will be more time for play and other physical contact. Take the long-term view. Your baby will be part of the family for years. Being patient and self-disciplined in the first few weeks can pay great dividends in establishing a workable family routine.

Patient comment

'Ryan'

The first four weeks of life with our baby Ryan made little difference to the normal routine of our first boy, aged 21 months. Ryan was breast-fed, slept, had a daily bath, several nappy changes, and many cuddles. More cuddles than his older brother had at that age. With our first child I was told I would 'spoil' him by 'too much handling', so as a newborn I only handled him as seemed necessary for his comfort. This time around I had been informed by more recent reading that I could not cuddle a newborn too much. I was delighted to take this advice.

Ryan was very placid and relaxed in his first four weeks. We hardly knew he was around. Suddenly he began waking up between feeds and crying, having only brief intervals of sleep and crying. His feeding behaviour was on and off suckling and crying, and he fell asleep before it seemed his hunger was fully satisfied. When laid down, his arms and legs seemed to tremble and twitch. Even when picked up, Ryan clenched his fist to his chest or under his chin and bore a worried expression. We decided his tension was from not enough cuddles—perhaps he felt insecure? We decided his perpetual waking was because he was not tired enough to sleep, and therefore his feeding behaviour was poor as he had not worked up an appetite while awake. I would like to point out that as our first child was a very sick baby we had no idea what 'normal' babies did. Hoping to help Ryan, we picked him up to calm him during crying periods and rewrapped him before laying him down. Then we would be awake perhaps 90 minutes or more at a time, cuddling and talking to him. He always went to bed in tears despite our efforts to make him feel better. For my husband and I this resulted in broken sleep getting only two to three hour sleep periods at best in a six to eight hour night. After several days of this we suffered headaches, and I was aware of having a hopeless memory and poor concentration for any task at all. Our firstborn's routine and behaviour was unaffected, but he did appear concerned for Ryan when he cried.

I sought advice. The following suggestions were made:

- Place a hot water bottle in the bassinet while feeding so that baby may return to a warm bed.
- Play a womb noises tape.
- Have the radio going near his bed through the night.
- Have baby sleep in our room during the night on my side of the bed, so that when he awoke during the night I had only to reach out and rock him back to sleep.

Really, I was amused and amazed. I could not in my practical mind take these suggestions seriously. Fortunately I had mentioned our problem to a friend who loaned me a copy of the book you are reading now. I actually read it from cover to cover on first reading. So much common sense, so much that made sense! Finally I turned to the Instant Diagnosis section and pin-pointed overtiredness as a common indicator and re-read the section on Presentation of Overtiredness. I felt that this was the problem, and after talking to my husband we decided to strictly follow the treatment as advised. That was difficult initially, but Ryan surprised us by transforming his behaviour within a few days.

We treated Ryan as follows:

- Using the crying down technique to a maximum of 10 minutes.
- Only handling Ryan during feeds and then for no more than a one-hour period.
- Carrying on our usual routine and allowing normal noise levels day and night.

The results within days were as follows:

- When being moved about, Ryan's limbs were relaxed and without twitches.
- Ryan fed placidly and well and remained awake throughout a 45–60 minute feed period.
- He routinely fed then slept throughout a 24 hour period with a minimum of being unsettled.
- Ryan slept for seven to ten hours a night from this time onwards.

Obviously, we settled down. Although two little boys are tiring, we now have enough sleep and enough peace to manage our days effectively and enjoyably.

K & MP

The first two years

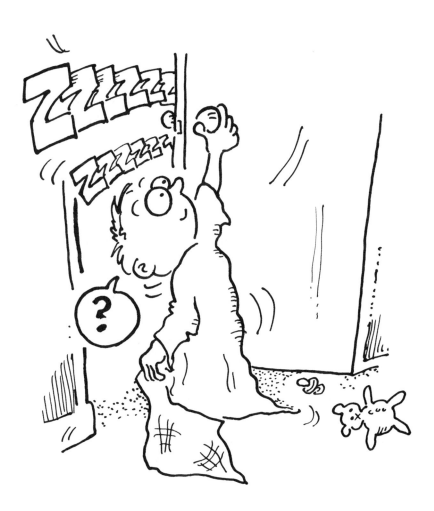

IN THE FOLLOWING description of the first two years of life, the order in which the information is presented is approximately related to age. Thus the first description usually relates to the youngest infant and the last description to the oldest. There will clearly be a large overlap between different children.

The behaviour of the overtired child

The following is a general description of some behaviour patterns which *may* be found in an overtired *child*. If your toddler gets tired but still behaves like an angel, then read no further. If you see a description of your child below, then at least part of the cause is probably tiredness.

Body language

In the very young child, say in the first year, the signs of tiredness can be subtle. Body posture can give some hints. The baby who is well rested, has a full stomach and is ready for sleep will often have a relaxed body posture. Her head tends to be on one side, eyes closed or closing, her arms are heavy and out straight. I sometimes describe these babies as being 'happy drunks' and most mothers recognise what I mean.

The opposite to this is the overtired baby. Her eyes are often open, her arms are flexed at the elbows, muscle tone is tight and she frequently cries. Her facial expression will often contain a little frown or scowl. Her hands often tremble. Some parents mistake this for shivering, but at the same time are confused as they know that the child is warm. The startle reflex is often very brisk. Sometimes even a loud noise can cause a reflex where the arms suddenly spread wide apart and then the hands come together towards the chest.

Interpreting these patterns is part of learning to 'read' your baby.

The eyes

There are two things to look at here. The first is what I refer to as 'meaningful eye contact'. This is difficult to put into words because it is an emotional event. When you look into the eyes of a healthy, well rested baby or child, there is a sense of emotional connection. Some exchange of emotion occurs. Parents and teachers never seem to hesitate when this idea is put to them. They know what is meant.

The reverse of meaningful eye contact is blank contact. You may lock eyes with your baby, but his expression is blank. No emotional exchange occurs. The child could be looking at a brick for all the response that you feel. As a child becomes increasingly tired, his ability to make meaningful eye contact decreases. If you are struggling with fatigue in your baby, then as his sleep improves, as he 'deposits more sleep into his sleep bank', one of the markers of success will be improved eye contact.

The second eye sign is deceptive and traps some parents. The eyes are wide open. People generally expect tiredness to lead to blinking or even closing of the eyes. While this is usually true, in the very overtired infant the reverse is the case. Watch carefully, and if your baby becomes badly over-tired his eyes may be wide open. The expression is often 'startled awake'. Sometimes the eyes will be so widely open that you will see the white of the eye above the iris. The trap here is that when the parents are discussing the problem, someone, quite logically, says 'He can't be tired, look at how wide open his eyes are.' Logical, but wrong. Beware of the tearful baby who only settles in your arms and in whom the eyes are 'startled open' a lot of the time. This child is likely to be severely overtired.

Security

The well rested infant gains emotional confidence, partly by being refreshed. While enjoying your company and touch, the child will not be overly distressed by being alone for reasonable periods of time. The child who needs to be in your arms or your lap may well be overtired. See the discussion of 'confidence radius' on page 140 for a more complete description.

Mood

Mood is a term that applies to every age. If any of us are overtired, it is difficult to be happy. As the child becomes more tired, smiles will be harder to get, shorter lived, and less frequent. Children who are rested are almost always happier and easier to live with.

Frustration tolerance

The overtired child will be annoyed at not getting her own way. Removing unsafe toys, turning off a tap, turning down the volume control on the TV—all are met with rage and irritability. Many of you will have seen Oscar-winning rages brought about by an action such as the removal of a biscuit. If the biscuit is returned, it is thrown away. You are now in a no-win situation. Getting angry simply raises the stakes and generally worsens the situation as the overtired child has gone past the point of reacting rationally to parental direction.

Achieve sleep as soon as possible. It is usually the only way forward.

Clumsy play

This one is easy. Overtired children play clumsily, tend to fall over or off things. They are often bumping into objects both stationary and mobile. This clumsiness reduces with better sleep. Some parents report that as the child's sleep improves, even after falling he is more tolerant of the discomfort and cries less. He gets up and plays with little fuss.

Eating

A small majority of the children that I see for the first visit have both feeding and sleeping problems. Of these the primary problem is usually sleep: fix the sleep and the diet often improves. It is not uncommon for parents to report that, even though their child was regarded as a good or adequate eater, after her sleep improved, her appetite did also.

The overtired, poor eater has the whole orchestra of common domestic feeding problems: inadequate volumes, inadequate range of foods, intermittent food refusal, and commonly a preference for drinks and milk drinks in particular. Parents often describe their children as grazing or browsing through the day.

For the majority of children in whom sleep is the primary problem, once sleep performance is improved and the child begins to achieve between ten and twelve hours sleep overnight, breakfast becomes an attractive proposition.

As a side issue, feeding problems in the 2 to 5 year age group can usually be resolved. Here are the basic steps I use in addressing feeding problems if they continue once the child is sleeping well.

- Food is not the issue. This is a power game. 'I will not do what you want because I wish to be in control.' Children at this age are not old enough to be given responsibility for their diets. If teenagers make a mess of it, imagine what a two-year-old would arrange! If the issue is power, and it is, take control and be confident at setting sensible, nutritionally appropriate, rules.

- Give solid foods before liquids. Give the cereal before the glass of milk.

- If the meal is not eaten well, do not become embroiled in a fight. Meal times are for eating, not fighting. Clear away the food, and send the child off to play. 'The next meal will be in four hours. By the way, there is nothing to eat or drink until the next meal.' Please take heart. It takes weeks to starve, but only a few hours to become seriously hungry. The trick here is to avoid 'snacks' between meals. Bring the child to the next meal hungry and thirsty.

- Be consistent. This is a power play. Once the child recognises that her parents are not a pushover and that your rules about eating are non negotiable, she will comply.

- At the end of the program, your child should be eating three meals per day where the volume of food, range of food, and speed of eating are consistent with the norms for your family.

Resolving sleep problems in the older child

Newborn babies are great in that they stay where you put them. By something between nine to 18 months children are mobile, and by the age of two years a lot of them can climb out of cots and open doors. The mobile, door-opening, bad sleeper is hard to ignore as he comes to you even if you won't go to him.

Sleep basics are the same as for other ages. Going to sleep is usefully regarded as a learned skill. Sleep achievement is partly based upon cues of sleep—the things or objects in the vicinity plus routines and styles of management. Cues of sleep are learned.

Almost universally in poor sleepers, one or other parent has become a necessary cue for sleep achievement and sleep maintenance. The task then is to allow the toddler to learn cues of sleep that are parent independent. Unfortunately, these children are hard to ignore because of their mobility. You may have a perfect program of sleep achievement, but at 2 a.m. there is the patter of little feet, or a little body sliding into the bed beside you. Some children perfect this technique to the stage that you do not hear or even feel them getting into bed. You just wake up at some time to realise that there is an extra body in the bed.

How do we handle this problem?

Bribing, rationalising, arguing and pleading will not work. For the child there is no greater reward than your company. (This appears not to be true for teenagers.) They are too young to realise that you deserve a good night's sleep. Anger is counter-productive, as it leads to insecurity and a greater need to obtain security by receiving affectionate contact from a parent.

So what works?

The answer sounds terrible and unloving, but once the child is mobile to the extent of getting out of a cot or bed and opening a door, we only have one choice. Secure the door. This will tug at your heart considerably, as it feels terrible to be 'locking' your child in her room. This advice is hard to give and hard to apply, but there is no other choice once the child is mobile. The positive side is that once applied consistently it is rapidly effective. In addition, all is forgiven once the family is sleeping well. Never has a family reported to me that they believed the experience led to emotional damage. Almost always parents report that both they and the children are happier with better sleep and that the improved quality of their relationships more than outweighs the cost of a couple of nights' crying.

The sequence of events from this point takes one of two broad paths.

Younger child less capable of verbal negotiation

The child is put to bed with a request to stay in bed or else the door will be closed and secured. As you leave the room, your child follows you out. So you return him to the bed or cot and leave, securing the door as you go. The child cries vigorously behind the door, demanding your return. You return and give minimal reassurance at 15, 20, 25, 30 minute intervals. The reassurance is short-lived and as simple as you can arrange. Thirty to sixty seconds of returning the child to the bed, a settling touch and a few words, and you go, securing the door behind you. Gradually increase the time that the child is alone until sleep is achieved. If sleep is achieved

on the floor either gently return him to bed, or, if this wakes
the child, gently cover him so that he will not become cold.
If the child wakes through the night, simply return him to
bed at once, secure the door and do no more until sleep is
achieved again. Check your child once you are sure he is
asleep. Repeat this every night until the child accepts that the
place for sleeping is in his own bed. As long as you are completely consistent, you should have major success within a
week. The door is then left open or closed as you see fit.

Older children able to negotiate verbally

With the older child of, say, two and a half years or above,
you can discuss the problem during the day. Some children
will even agree with you that yes, they are big boys and girls
now, and yes they can sleep through the night alone. Of
course, come nightfall all is forgotten and the sleep disturbances begin again. You have forewarned your child about
the door and so you now lock it and go through the program
of diminishing reassurance described above.

The difference here is that the older child will negotiate.
Commonly she will offer an alternative to the locked
door: 'Dad, if you leave the door open I will stay in bed.'
Unfortunately, as soon as the door is open all promises are
cancelled and you have company again.

The key here is the response. The child is instantly
returned to bed. Try to remain even-tempered because you
certainly have the upper hand now. Return her to bed and
lock the door until sleep is achieved. No variation of your
plan, which you both negotiated, is allowed. This approach
seems to work rapidly, and it appears to lead to independent
sleep in something between four and seven nights. Any break-
down in the child's adhering to the rules immediately leads
to a return to bed and securing the door.

A *word of warning*

Make sure the bedroom is childproof. Some children will empty drawers, take down pictures, kick doors, ride rocking horses, and generally be imaginative in expressing their opinion about Dr Symon's advice.

Patient comment

'Matthew'

> At seven months, our son's nocturnal routine was to wake just before midnight. He would cry and scream until we could pick him up and then he would miraculously fall asleep in our arms, only to wake up again when placed in his cot. We had tried wrapping, rocking, a night light, a roll-over feed and nursing, but nothing seemed to work consistently.
>
> We got to the stage that Matthew would end up in bed with my husband and I. It was something we didn't want, but we both agreed that we had no choice. Each night was survival of the fittest, and the most frustrating and exhausting thing was that Matthew was fitter than both of us.
>
> Dr Symon came into our nightly fiasco after we questioned the sedative approach another doctor recommended. He explained sleeping, my son's pattern of sleep, and that it was possible to teach Matthew to sleep and to sleep 12 hours every night.
>
> His technique was very basic, although one had to be committed and to know that we were on the way to a child that slept well. We gained the confidence that as parents we were capable of teaching Matthew how to fall asleep by himself and to go back to sleep should he wake up.
>
> My relationship with my husband certainly benefited from Matthew sleeping consistently during the night. Each morning we wanted to see him and didn't wake up frustrated and tired because he had kept us up during the night.

Matthew is certainly a happy, loving and eager 10-month-old boy. I'm sure it is mainly due to his sleeping well.

His parents are sleeping too. Friends label us as 'lucky' to have a child who sleeps. We confidently know and explain that we had a 'sleep doctor' who taught us how to teach Matthew to sleep when he needed to.

Day sleep

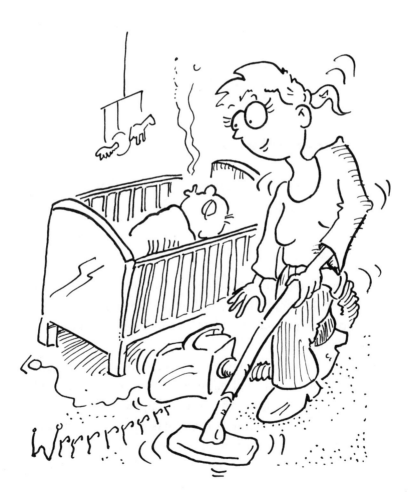

WHILE THE VAST majority of parents come to see me about night-time sleep problems, daytime sleep problems are often harder to solve. This is not such a severe problem for the parents in that it is possible to be far more patient and forgiving during the day once your child's night sleep has improved and you are sleeping well overnight.

I find it useful to divide sleep periods into three groups: night, morning, and afternoon. While the night is usually the biggest problem for families it is the one area which improves most rapidly. The morning is next to improve. The most difficult time of day to achieve good control of an infant's sleep performance is the afternoon. Remember that while this is generally true, your baby may be different. He may not have read this book.

Daytime advice

The advice about daytime sleep is similar to that for the night but with a couple of minor variations.

Happy wake times

The key to daytime success is a concept which I call the 'happy wake time'. Happy wake time is a simple yet powerful tool in your understanding and management of daytime sleep disorders.

Imagine your child having slept well overnight. She wakes in a good mood. (It will happen, I promise.) She is hungry, and once fed is happy. She is in a 'happy wake time'. The key to a happy wake time is that it has a beginning, a middle and an end. The *end* of the happy wake time is announced by changes in the child's behaviour. She begins to rub at her eyes, to whimper, to seek out your company for support or to become grizzly in the number of little ways which you will come to recognise rapidly and accurately.

This is the time to put her down. This is the time when she is best able to achieve sleep. With every half hour that passes beyond this point, the child is going further into *overtired* time. The more overtired the child becomes the more difficult it is for her to get to sleep, to perform the learned skill of achieving sleep efficiently.

Many of the parents I see are missing the end of the happy wake time and allowing their child to become overtired. She then has trouble achieving sleep and cries vigorously. The parents then lose confidence in their decision that the child was tired and needed to go down. The baby is then lifted up, settled in the parents' arms, but becomes increasingly tired and grizzly and less able to achieve sleep efficiently. A common time for this is the afternoon. One of my families described 5 p.m. as suicide hour.

The key advice here is as follows. When you know that the baby is well, has had enough to eat and has reached the end of her happy wake time, then put her down and allow her the chance to achieve sleep alone. If you pick the time accurately she will achieve sleep efficiently. The more tired the child becomes, the more she needs sleep, the more tearful she may become while sleep is being achieved.

Remember it is only appropriate to ignore the crying baby when she is well, gaining weight correctly, and no other cause for distress exists.

How long are happy wake times?

This question has multiple answers. Generally, the happy wake time is shorter than most people expect. For example, a baby of twelve weeks who is sleeping well overnight may be tired and ready for another sleep of two or three hours after only one to one and a half hours of being awake. The shortest happy wake times tend to be early in the day. This appears illogical as the child has just had his longest sleep. Despite the lack of logic, that is how things work. The baby's own behaviour is the best indicator of the length of the happy wake time.

A baby who is sleeping well and receiving adequate food is generally in a good mood. As he becomes tired his mood deteriorates. He becomes more tearful, seeks out parental care more, is less emotionally independent, plays for shorter times with one object, and is more likely to be destructive in his play. Use your child's behaviour as the guide to the length of waking time which is appropriate.

Blended behaviour

Blended behaviour is a concept I find helpful for parents who are confused by their children's behaviour.

Imagine that a child's behaviour is divided into two styles only: happy and well, and tired and 'scratchy'. This is simplistic, but it works.

As the child becomes more overtired these two patterns of behaviour blend. She becomes harder to 'read'. You think that she is tired and then she gives you a big smile. At another time you believe that she is well and happy, but her smile will suddenly change to loud inconsolable crying for no obvious reason. This 'blended behaviour' is a catch for the unwary. It can leave you confused and desperate in trying to understand your baby. Once you recognise it for what it is, you are a long way towards getting control of the situation. Blended behaviour is most commonly a result of fatigue. The child wants to be cheerful and loving but is just too tired to put it together consistently. The solution is obvious: more sleep.

Sleep achievement in the day

For night sleep I advocate a program of minimal reassurance. The baby or child receives less and less contact with you as sleep is achieved. As you gain confidence the child is left alone for longer and longer periods to achieve sleep.

For day sleep the advice is similar, but differs slightly.

Once you have decided that it is time for sleep, go through your normal pre-sleep pattern. Place the child in his cot or bed and settle him as you normally would. To the best of your ability, leave him to achieve sleep alone. If he protests, then depending on his age leave him alone for between 5 and 15 minutes.

For this discussion let's assume that you leave the child to protest for 10 minutes. After 10 minutes you return and reassure the baby with a little touch—perhaps resupply the dummy—a few kind words, and then leave. Avoid patting, rocking, holding or other styles of reassurance which include prolonged parental care. If the protests continue, return after 15 minutes and repeat the short reassurance. This may be repeated again after another 20 minutes. If this has failed then the child has been protesting for at least 45 minutes. At night I advocate that you just continue. During the day the advice is different. During daylight hours I set an upper limit of 45 minutes of crying. The reason for this is that it is too harsh on the parent who is listening to the child's cries. Some children will cry for a couple of hours, particularly if they have become overtired. If I ask a mother or father to listen to this crying for hours it becomes distressing and can lead to a loss of confidence. Because of this I allow the baby to be lifted after 45 minutes. This time is approximately equal to one sleep cycle. The child is lifted and fed, reassured and settled.

Despite this compromise it is important to recognise that you were almost definitely correct that the baby needed sleep 45 minutes previously. The child is now tired plus 45 minutes of protest. His ability to be usefully awake is thus limited. Allow him to settle, but as soon as you see the signs of tiredness appearing return him to his place of sleep and repeat the process. The baby may only be up for 30 to 60 minutes before you are deciding that it is time for sleep again. Keep on cycling in this way until sleep is achieved.

Remember that morning sleeps will improve before afternoon sleeps in most children.

Conclusion

- Daytime sleep requires just as much attention as night sleep.
- Use the concept of the happy wake time to choose when the child is ready for sleep.
- Avoid the child becoming overtired. Increasing levels of fatigue will interfere with her ability to achieve sleep. Put the child down sooner rather than later.
- Once you know that the child is ready for sleep, go through your normal preparations for bedtime and then leave the child *alone* to achieve sleep.
- During the day I generally recommend a maximum of one sleep cycle of protest and then allow the child to come out of the cot and to be settled in the parents' company.

- If the baby is demonstrating 'blended behaviour'
  then there is almost definitely a need for more sleep
  to be achieved.
- Do not be discouraged if you have good control at
  night and it takes longer to achieve satisfactory control
  of the day. That is normal.

Dreams and nightmares

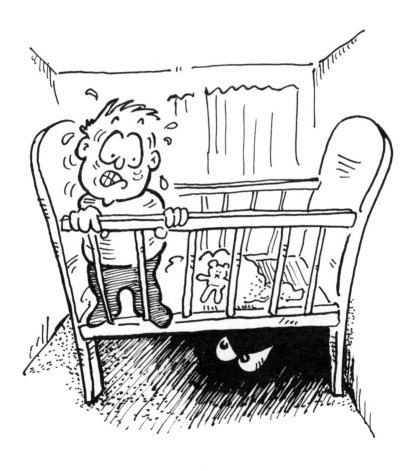

MANY PARENTS ATTEMPTING to achieve independent sleep for their children face the problem of 'nightmares'. These are sometimes clearly described by the children. They may include spiders under the bed, monsters in the cupboard, robbers at the door, or my favourite: 'teddy will get me during the night'. The oldest patient that I have seen who was disturbed by dreams was ten years old. Her parents were getting up about three times per night to protect her from robbers at the door. (I will return to this patient in a little while.) Sometimes the dreams are not clearly described and the diagnosis of nightmares is made by the parents, based upon their opinions of the child's 'style of distress' during the night.

Before addressing the question of nightmares, it is worthwhile talking about dreams.

Do young children dream?

Dreaming occurs in a stage of sleep known as rapid eye movement sleep or REM sleep. Children certainly have REM sleep. In fact, the younger the child the more REM sleep that occurs, and the earlier in a block of sleep that it begins. In the first six months of life the infant moves straight into REM sleep, whereas adults enter NREM sleep first.

REM sleep is a time of much brain activity and, for the young child, much body movement. Those who have slept with an infant will probably have noticed the very vigorous way in which they sleep. One mother described it to me as sleeping with a little tornado. As REM sleep in adults is our time of dreaming and this sleep phase is identifiable in babies and children, it would appear reasonable to assume that children also 'dream' in this phase of their sleep if they are able to.

The next question is: what do they dream about? It is of no value to discuss the content of the dreams for the very young baby as we have no way of checking with the baby.

The child who is able to talk may report the content of his dreams. The youngest child I have encountered who could talk about dreaming was 18 months old. He was a boy who had developed communication skills very early in life and would report clearly on his thoughts. He reported that his dreams contained the stuff of dreams which we would probably predict. He dreamt of toys and play animals, of family members, of Mickey Mouse and Donald Duck. The evidence here was that a child as early as 18 months is having dreams that clearly connect with his life experience.

Nightmares are a variety of dreams where the content of the thought process includes fear, anxiety or terror. As we all know, such dreams can interfere with our sleep, and cause us to wake in fear.

Are nightmares relevant to childhood sleep? Are they a possible explanation for night-time waking in tears? The answer here will be divided into two ages: the very young child, and the older infant with verbal skills.

Nightmares in the very young child (birth to 12 months)

It is difficult to conceive that a child has nightmares at this age.

The infant brain is at an early stage of development and is beginning the process of learning how to interpret the environment meaningfully. At the same time the child's brain is developing rapidly to be capable of 'thinking' in a way which is meaningful.

I do not wish to become embroiled in a discussion here

where no matter what is argued it is nearly impossible to prove the existence of nightmares. My own belief is that nightmares do not occur at this age. This is based upon a belief that the infant brain is not yet able to process information in such a complex way.

Whatever the situation, I can predict one thing from experience. It is useful to *assume* that if the child is crying it is *not* due to nightmares. Excluding nightmares as a diagnosis removes one more problem the parents could worry about.

Nightmares in the older child (18 months plus)

As mentioned above, I have spoken to a child who could report on his dreams as early as 18 months of age. Thus the child at this age is now able to coordinate recognisable thought processes while in REM sleep.

If nightmares are possible, I then divide them into two groups: real and relevant, and real but not relevant.

Real and relevant

An infant's thoughts will reflect his life experience. If that experience includes fear, anxiety, or anger, then that may be reflected in nightmares. Such unhappy daytime experience will almost always be known to the family. If home life contains anger, fighting or instability, then this may be a cause of insecurity resulting in disturbed sleep.

These problems need to be addressed as family problems, not as sleep disorders. My advice about sleep will not be useful or appropriate in this setting.

Children of an older age, say school age, may begin to

have nightmares reflecting problems with their peers. This again needs to be diagnosed and treated on its merits.

Real but not relevant

The 'real but not relevant' group occurs most frequently. It is an area where the game of life can be played between parent and child. Irrelevant nightmares can be a powerful tool for a young, talkative child to use in controlling parental behaviour. It is also an area in which parents must recognise what is happening because there are dangers in *allowing* a child to have nightmares.

This seems a strange concept. To explain, let me tell you a story. I have seen a girl of ten years, whom I will call Angela. Her parents brought her to see me because of a sleep disorder. She was up, or more to the point, *they* were up, three times a night on average. After ten years it was all wearing a little thin. This was not a happy family. Angela herself was bright, cheerful, talkative, and obviously thriving. (Her parents were still talking. Just.) It quickly became apparent that Angela was waking her family at night because of 'the robbers'. There were robbers at the door or the window every night. In fact they had been calling, regularly, every night for about eight years. Angela would wake and cry, one of her parents would come to her aid, turn on the light, prove the absence of any thief, and return to bed. Most nights one of her parents would finally sleep with Angela, or in her room, or on a mattress made ready for the purpose outside their daughter's room.

The problem was obviously not robbers, but the belief in robbers. This belief structure had existed for eight years. Why? How do these thoughts arise?

It all begins in that time, let's say about age two years, when verbal skills are beginning to develop. For some reason, the child is up during the night and quite logically seeking contact with her parents. The parents do a check that all is well and attempt to return their child to bed. The child is now old enough and bright enough to offer some alternatives.

'I want a drink.'

'I need to go to the toilet.'

'I'm hungry.'

These are neutral requests which are easily ignored or complied with. If you want to be getting up to provide your children with a drink of milk for a few months, just start. Your children will be quite happy to continue to push the button for room service until the night staff eventually quit.

Other requests can be more subtle and demanding.

'I'm scared.'

'There's a monster in the cupboard.'

'There's a spider under the bed.'

The problem here is that you feel a logical and appropriate desire to reassure your child that she is safe. This rewards the behaviour pattern of reporting the 'monster'. Next night you feel less inclined to be reassuring and you try to dismiss the claim with 'There's no monster'. The child is then obliged to amplify her level of fear to obtain the reward of your company. She appears even more anxious than the night before. The 'fear' becomes worse. Most parents eventually get tired of the game, stop attending, or give minimal reassurance. The fear is then not being rewarded, has less relevance, and then stops. Unfortunately, for a few families, the child's state of fear becomes dramatic enough for the parents to continue giving reassurance. This continues to reward the holding of a state of fear. Being scared becomes an unconscious but useful strategy for the child.

One of the complicating factors here is that because the

state of fear is useful, it becomes more complex. As the weeks and months go by, the state of anxiety develops more depth and realism. It can, occasionally, become permanent or semi-permanent. While none of this is conscious or planned, these 'imagined' problems can become a regular night-time event. Unfortunately once the state of fear becomes so real at night, it can begin to affect the days.

Let's return to Angela's story.

For years Angela had found that she could successfully obtain parental attention at night by reporting with great anguish that the robbers were at the windows. While she was bright and happy in her family circle, she became timid of certain public areas in the day. She was hesitant to walk unaccompanied because 'someone from the robbers' might get her. The fear had become so real that it interfered with her daytime activities.

The moral of the story is that night-time fears that are obviously without foundation need to be dismissed as rapidly as possible. Rewarding unfounded night-time fears leads to those fears being prolonged.

How should we handle inappropriate nightmares or night fears?

The first step is to check on the reality. Is there really a spider on the floor? (Don't spend too much time on checking the monster in the cupboard.) Once you are satisfied that the fear is not caused by a real problem, but has been generated in an attempt to control your behaviour, then ignore it. If at all possible, try to avoid becoming angry; simply recognise that your child loves you, has woken at night, and is attempting either to generate contact with you or to prolong it. Recognise it for what it is, and politely decline to participate in the life story of the monster in the cupboard. Once you fail to respond, the monster has no value, and goes away.

A little hint. I sometimes ask the child in the consulting room to draw me a picture of the monster, or prompt me in drawing one. Once we have agreed that this picture is correct, I keep it. The parents can then tell the child, 'Don't be scared. Dr Symon kept the monster.' This sometimes works rapidly.

To conclude Angela's story. Because of her intelligence and age, I was able to explain the history of the robbers to her and her parents. She could see the logic of it but was left with an involuntary fear state which woke her. The solution was achieved using the following elements.

Her parents were not to respond. (Remove the reward.)

When Angela was woken by fear, she was allowed to take control of her room. She locked the door, which made her feel safer. She was allowed to put on a light and read, which she loved. She had a torch to shine at the window to prove to herself that no robbers were present.

Angela was able to sleep a full night two weeks after starting. She didn't miss the robbers. Her parents enjoyed the increased sleep, and family life has improved dramatically.

Angela was kind enough to agree to write a little about her experience. She typed the summary herself, in her own words.

Angela's comments on sleep

Dr Symon made me feel like I wasn't a baby when I had my sleeping problem. And he made me realise that it was just in my head. It was just my brain playing tricks on me; my mind playing games. And when I heard noises, I just pushed it out of my mind, remembering what Dr Symon had said: 'It's just my imagination. It's just my brain playing up.'

One night I heard lots of noises and then in the morning nothing was gone and my mum was sleeping in the lounge room where the noises had come from. So it had to be my imagination—my brain playing with me.

It's helped me because it has made everyone in my family a lot more cheerful. Now I am happy that I can sleep through the night and not worry every time I go to bed. Now I know I can go back to sleep if I wake up in the middle of the night. Now sometimes I wake up three or four times a night and can still go back to sleep. Before I was always worried at bedtime because I would wake up in the middle of the night, hear noises, get VERY scared and not be able to get back to sleep on my own. NOW I CAN!

Before I could not sleep over at friend's houses, but now I feel a lot safer and I can do it. I went on camp and didn't get scared once! (It was a two-night camp.) At the beginning of the year my mum and dad thought I'd never be able to go on camp and didn't want to pay the money for camp. But I DID IT!!

Angela's parents informed me that these two examples of sleeping over and attending a camp were the first successful nights away in her life.

In conclusion on nightmares

For the young child, say younger than twelve months, it is most useful to assume that nightmares do not occur. For the child from 18 months up, nightmares should be divided into two groups.

The first group is nightmares that reflect daytime un-happiness or insecurity. If family problems exist, these will need attention in the first instance. Sleep performance will not improve while there is a genuine reason for being insecure and awake overnight.

The second group is nightmares or fear states that are simply a tool for controlling parental behaviour. These need to be deleted as rapidly as possible. Inappropriate dreams are deleted by not responding to them.

Night terrors

'Night terrors' is an unfortunate term, as it suggests a problem which may not be present. Despite this, the use of the term is so common that it needs to be discussed.

'Night terrors' fall into two groups.

The first are the inappropriate fears that occur in the child who is old enough to talk and describe specific fears. These children need to be reassured and their fears played down and ignored as rapidly as possible, as is discussed above.

The second group is inappropriate awakenings. Waking up from sleep is a complex event that sometimes occurs incorrectly. The child is awake but confused, incoherent, makes no meaningful eye contact, often pushes the parent away, and is basically inconsolable. The best solution is to wrap or lay the child down. Reassure the child, to the best of your ability, even though it appears to be ineffective, and leave him alone. Let him get to sleep again as rapidly as possible. Another possible solution is full awakening. I do not recommend this, as you are then left with the problem of a return to sleep anyway. These night terrors become less frequent as the child's sleep improves.

Both of these sleep disturbances can be worrying for the parents. Both are better controlled by a minor reaction from parents than a major reaction.

Winning

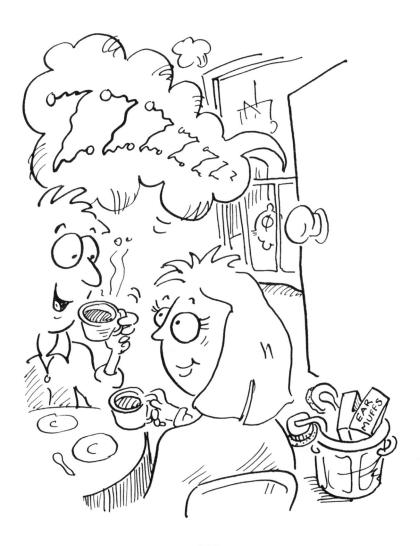

EVERY CHILD IS UNIQUE, and every family is different and does things in its own way. So in talking about sleep problems and teaching sleep skills, there is always the danger of generalising in a way that is inappropriate for some or even many families. Despite this, changes that occur in children as their sleep improves are remarkably consistent. I will outline events that commonly occur.

Having decided to regain control of the child's sleep routine for the sanity or even the survival of the family, you begin to implement the plan described in this book. There are four main phases in the improvement: protest, rapid improvement, negotiation, and behavioural improvement.

Protest

The aim of this program is to enable the child to learn independent skills of sleep achievement. Almost always this involves removing the parents from the actual time of sleep transition. Now, as far as the child is concerned, her mother is the most attractive, most needed woman in the world, and her father is the most wonderful man. When you are removed from the moment of sleep achievement, your child will, quite logically, have an adverse opinion. As you leave the bedroom, she will almost certainly protest loudly. This also is logical and easily understood. I generally suggest to my patients that the child is complaining about the wicked doctor; that they, the child and the parent, had a much better system, and that mum, or dad, should return at once and keep on doing what has been normal for months.

Your child's protest is logical, understandable, and loud. It tugs at your heart. It needs to be ignored in a way that helps to develop sleep skills. I won't repeat the program of decreased handling here; see Chapter 4, Sleep Problems, for a full description.

The good news is that the protests will decrease in a fairly predictable way. I say 'fairly', because there is a big range in the way children respond to the program.

About 10 per cent of children will cry briefly for 10 to 15 minutes, and then sleep for the rest of the night. I well remember a woman who saw me after 18 months of badly disrupted sleep. She applied this program and, on the first night, her child cried for 15 minutes and then slept for twelve hours. He then just slept each night thereafter. To my surprise, the mother was moderately annoyed by all this. 'Why hadn't someone told her about this before?' I think she did smile at me a little as she left.

A small minority of children will improve very quickly. A small minority will improve very slowly. (For more information on this group, see Chapter 12, Failure.) The majority of children will be in the middle, and their protests will decrease fairly rapidly.

If your child can't speak yet, jump now to the next section. If your child is old enough to talk and negotiate, then read on. Slightly older children have some interesting little tricks.

While a child is very young, she can only cry. The talkative toddler can do more than cry. The child can now imagine, make excuses, and negotiate. She will often have a fertile imagination and, despite your best intentions, will always be one step ahead. Remember the child has only one objective during the night and that is to maximise contact time with her parents. Whatever you do to meet one of her demands and let her return to sleep, will therefore never be quite right. If her mother is present, she may ask for her father. If her father is present, she may want her mother. The range of requests is never ending. 'I want a drink.' 'I want to eat.'

'I need to go to the toilet.' 'I'm cold.' 'I'm hot.' As rapidly as you meet one need, another will appear. The most worrying are anxieties and terrors. For a longer discussion of this, see Chapter 9, Dreams and Nightmares.

The rule to remember is that your child, whom you love and who loves you, is simply protesting at a new style of sleep achievement which excludes parental contact. Independent sleep carries so many advantages for the whole family that every endeavour must be made to ignore these attempts at negotiation. If your child is well, properly fed and clothed, and if the time is appropriate for sleep, then politely but firmly decline to become embroiled in these efforts at negotiation. You need to be in charge of the night, not your offspring. She will protest, but trust me, the future is bright. Read on.

Rapid improvement

Once a program of teaching independent sleep skills is commenced, progress is *usually* (but not always) rapid. There are variations from child to child and family to family.

The two major variables that affect the rate of improvement are fatigue, and consistency.

Fatigue

Remember that we are teaching a skill. In this setting it is the skill of making the transition from wakefulness to sleep independently of parental contact. Like any new skill, this is harder to learn if the child is severely overtired. The more severe the sleep problem, the slower the improvement. This is an area of parental confusion because, as adults, we think of sleep achievement as being driven by tiredness. It is only when we regard sleep achievement as a learned process that the negative impact of fatigue becomes logical.

Consistency

Once begun, the training program must be consistent. There are major problems with an inconsistent approach, such as teaching 'persistent crying behaviour'. This is discussed at length in Chapter 11, Losing It.

With a loving but consistent approach, children will achieve more hours of sleep. As they achieve more rest, their ability to learn the new skills of sleep achievement, and put them into practice, rapidly improves.

Many families report at their second visit, 'If only we had known how effective it would be, we would have done this months ago.'

Rapid improvement needs further explanation.

Children will protest vigorously at the removal of a parental figure from the time of their sleep achievement. It is difficult to predict how much crying or calling out a specific child will produce, but the rate of improvement has a degree of predictability. The child's protests will often decrease at a rate of about 50 per cent per night or better. There will be variation depending upon specific circumstances, but the crying on the second night is often 50 per cent less than the first. The third night is often 50 per cent better again, or 25 per cent of the first night's effort. It is not unusual for long blocks of sleep to be achieved by the third, fourth, or fifth night. For parents who have been up many times a night for months, this may seem like rapid improvement. A full night's sleep is a very rewarding experience.

Having said this, there is a trap which I will call negotiation. The phase of negotiation is a trap for the unwary and unprepared.

Negotiation

It is one of life's little axioms that if you are really having a nice day, something will try to trip you up. In our case, if you have started to enjoy a full night's sleep, you may find there will be an attempt to return to the previous poor sleep behaviour.

In the sleep literature, where academics talk to academics, there is an event called the post-extinction reaction burst. In normal language, the infant has had a sleep problem, the parents start a program to improve sleep, the sleep does begin to improve, and then it seems to go wrong. The child who has begun to sleep for long blocks at night begins to wake again. This can be a major setback for the parents, and for some it marks the point of final surrender. 'We tried so hard for seven nights. It seemed to be working. Now listen to that cry. I've got to sleep or I'll be useless at work tomorrow. Let's get him up, bring him to our bed, and get some sleep.'

This phase is significant, and I call it the negotiation phase. What appears to happen is that the child who has been using the parent as a major cue for sleep achievement begins to sleep through after a period of decreasing protest. He achieves reasonable blocks of sleep and then something occurs in the child's subconscious to try it again. I describe it to families as a final effort to see if the parents really mean it, and are quite certain that they wouldn't like to come back for a cuddle at say two or three in the morning. This is the child's last subconscious effort to modify your behaviour back to the style of sleep that you saw as a problem in the first case. The rational response to this phase of negotiation is to see it for what it is. The baby or infant is asking, in his own way, 'Could you please come in and visit me now. I like it when you do.'

To comply with this request simply reinstates parent-dependent cues of sleep and so undoes the work of the preceding days and nights. The parents' response needs to be along these lines: 'Sorry darling, I feel much better when I've had a whole night's sleep. In fact, you were a much happier child today after last night's good sleep. I love you dearly, but night is for sleeping, I'm not coming'.

To the best of your ability, stay in bed. Ignore this attempt to negotiate, and allow your child to return to sleep alone. You may choose to check that the baby is well and safe, after you believe that he is asleep again.

The negotiation phase is random and difficult to predict. I cannot say on which night it will occur, or at what times the child will cry out. Simply recognise it for what it is, and don't become involved. Once this attempt to negotiate is ignored successfully, the child has completed the three initial phases of improvement and has now developed independent skills of sleep achievement and maintenance.

Behavioural improvement

Once good sleep is achieved, there are a number of areas that many parents report as improved. We know as parents that when we become overtired, there are consequences we don't like in our own behaviour. Many of us become short-tempered, forgetful, confused, and unaffectionate. Children also reflect the consequences of tiredness in many ways. Often their play is too boisterous or destructive, their concentration span may be poor, and their frustration tolerance may not exist. They become increasingly emotionally dependent, but at the same time less loving. Having said all this, there are certainly many children who cope very admirably with broken sleep, and who are loving, cheerful, and a joy to be with during the day. In these families, it is usually the parents who benefit from the improved sleep. Despite this, the majority of sleep-deprived children will be affected in some way that family or friends recognise. There are a number of typical signs of improvement.

Happiness

A child who has slept well overnight will usually wake happy. She may be hungry, but she is content. I generally expect the child who has achieved the amount of sleep she needs to wake quietly, patiently wait for her mother or father to come, and then greet them with obvious happiness and enthusiasm. This improved happiness will continue throughout the day until she starts to become tired.

Calmness

A well-rested child is calm. His play tends to be less intrusive and more constructive. He is more enjoyable to be with.

Concentration span

Once the child's mind and body are rested, parents will often report that she plays for longer periods with specific toys, or shows signs of being more focused on a task. Any adults who have been severely overtired will be able to relate to this improved ability to concentrate.

Frustration tolerance

Overtired children who are not getting their own way will often give an impressive display of temper. They throw themselves down on the ground, kick and scream. Older infants may turn on others and kick or bite or throw things. Attempts at negotiating with these children are useless, as they are usually past the point of responding to a 'reasonable' approach from the care giver. Many of you will have seen such children in the shopping mall giving their tired parents a terrible time, yelling and screaming. They are generally regarded as naughty or poorly behaved, but almost always it is simply fatigue. They have become too tired and are unable to accept not getting their own way.

The reverse occurs when sleep improves. Within a few days, behaviour becomes more logical, tolerance of frustration improves, and it becomes easier to talk the child into an alternative activity without screams of temper.

Having said this, beware of the end of the day. Even the child who is sleeping well still gets tired and may become testing before bedtime.

Affection

Another behaviour affected by fatigue is the giving of affection. Giving and receiving appropriate affection are the true rewards of parenthood. There are few feelings more satisfying than to be holding an infant who is loving and thriving. It is wonderful to receive unconditional love from your child. This is often shared by touching and holding.

An overtired child has trouble being affectionate. He is often dependent. He looks for your company, seeking contact, but when you hold him it is often a relationship of dependency. The child needs you and takes affection from you. Being in your arms is safe. There are many occasions where this behaviour is totally appropriate, but when it is too frequent it becomes wearing.

As children improve their sleep, their relationship with care givers and parents often becomes richer. At the same time, the quality and style of physical interaction improves. When the child is in your arms, he not only takes love, but gives it in return. It is heart-warming and strengthening to feel your child snuggle into your body and give affection to you. It may be a wet and clumsy kiss, but it's a kiss. This two-way emotional traffic is no longer draining and tiresome, but strengthening. If your sleep has improved as well, your chance of returning that affection is greater. When it begins to happen, particularly if you are coming from a background of months of tiredness and broken nights, you will know that you are heading in the right direction.

Confidence radius

In recent years, I have developed the concept of a 'confidence radius', which has proved to be a useful idea. Like so much in this book, it is simple but fairly widely applicable. The confidence radius is a distance which you can think of as metres or yards, although I never measure it as such because it is not necessary. Think of it as the distance between the carer and the child.

As children become tired, their ability to function away from a parental figure decreases. At the most extreme, the child will only be content resting in her parent's arms. As soon as an attempt is made to put the child down, she cries and becomes distressed. Slightly older children who are mobile will cry and follow you around the house. Their ability to feel confident alone is severely limited.

As children's sleep improves, so does their confidence. Once children are sleeping well, they become more comfortable in their own company. The general picture here is of a child who has slept well overnight, eaten breakfast of either milk or solids depending upon age, and is now happily awake. This child generally can be expected to enjoy the company of the care giver but will not become distressed if left alone. It should be possible to leave the room to attend to other responsibilities and for the child to be able to entertain herself with toys or mobiles or other appropriate activities.

This concept is a useful marker of fatigue. If your child is usually confident in a room alone, and over a day or two you notice that you are being called back more and more rapidly, then she is possibly becoming overtired. Conversely, if your child becomes less tired, you will notice an increase in her confidence radius.

Emotional independence and the ability to give affection are complementary. In some ways they may appear to be opposites, but they are two sides of the one coin.

Readability

The concept of readability connects with that of 'blended behaviour'. Overtired children can be difficult to read or interpret. Are they happy or sad? It is confusing for parents caring for an overtired child.

This can be simplified into behaviour patterns of two types. The first is that of overtiredness often associated with difficult behaviour. Rested behaviour is usually the reverse. The rested child is usually pleasant to be with, his play is not intrusive, his appetite tends to be good, he is more logical and consistent. Looking after him is a pleasure.

I often see children in whom prolonged tiredness leads

to a blending of these two styles of behaviour. Minutes of laughing and happy behaviour are mixed with minutes of unhappiness and difficult behaviour. In this setting, the parent may have trouble judging their child. The child may become difficult to 'read'. 'Is my child tired or not?'

Improved sleep leads to improved readability. The rested child is far more likely to be content. As normal tiredness develops during the day, it declares itself as a change in behaviour. Common signs include yawning, heavy blinking, rubbing at eyes, pulling an ear, or crying and whimpering. The child is tired but not overtired. If this tiredness is recognised quickly, and the child is put down for the next sleep, he is far more likely to achieve sleep efficiently.

One of the benefits of improved readability is that it increases your confidence that you understand what is happening and can take control. Those of you who think you have never been in control can take heart: things should improve soon.

Sleep-seeking behaviour

Sleep-seeking behaviour is a sign that parents have reported to me and it appears to be the final sign of success in teaching sleep skills. It only applies to the toddler and older child, and you will quickly understand why.

Recognising our own tiredness is one of the functions of the mind that we take for granted as adults. Some of you may feel that you are living in a permanent state of tiredness. Feeling exhausted is not fun, but understanding and recognising that you are tired is important. It is a function of self-care that we recognise our tiredness and take the necessary steps to fix the problem. To the best of our ability we plan and seek sleep. It is a sign of maturity to assume responsibility for our sleep.

Young children do not have an ability to recognise fatigue or make a decision to go to sleep. As the child matures she will at some stage begin to monitor herself and recognise tiredness. The magic moment for parents is when the child takes that extra step of development and recognises the solution. 'I'm tired. I need to sleep.'

When your toddler begins to report to you that she is tired, the battle is almost won. Once both you and your child recognise fatigue for what it is and that the solution to these feelings is sleep, then you are finally working together.

Patient comment

When we began our consultations, our 19-month-old son was not sleeping in the evening until 9 p.m., and then only after a lot of difficulty. Occasionally he would be awake until 9.30 or 10 p.m. He would wake up regularly during the night and usually ended up in bed with us. He would then wake at 6 a.m. He would not sleep in the afternoon unless he was rocked in our arms, with the duration of his nap being 40 minutes.

We followed 'the plan'. Within days we achieved a more reasonable sleep time in the evening. The nightly waking ceased a few days after we settled his evening routine. The afternoon nap was the most difficult routine to achieve, as our son had always been rocked in our arms and was very determined not to let go of this. We had to persevere, knowing it was to our son's benefit to achieve sleep by himself, at all times of the day or night.

Our son is now in bed at around 7 p.m. and content to go to sleep. He no longer wakes during the night and his day continues to start between 6.00 and 6.30 a.m. We are able to put him down for an afternoon nap, without any rocking, when he sleeps, on average, two hours. He is now a happier, less stressed and less stressful little boy.

Losing it

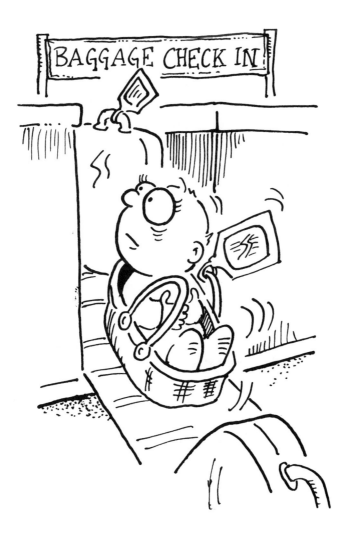

THERE IS SOMETHING wonderful about achieving a full night's sleep after weeks, months, or even years of broken sleep. It is not uncommon for people to come to a second consultation and say, 'Thank you, I've got my life back.' Family life improves; memory starts to function again. Some parents report that they have learned to talk to each other again, having spent months where the whole evening was devoted to child care and attempting to get a reluctant, over-tired child to sleep. In that setting, when the child does achieve good sleep routines, the parents suddenly find time for each other.

And then, sometimes, the child's sleep pattern crumbles again. Nights start to be disrupted, and the tiredness returns. Losing what was so dearly won is not fun.

'Losing it' can be devastating to your confidence. There are a number of events that can cause loss of routine. Almost always, you will clearly understand the cause. The more common causes include illness, moving house, moving inter-state or overseas, and daylight saving. I will deal with these in no particular order.

The information below and the guidelines for teaching sleep skills explained elsewhere in this book will usually be your lifeline back to normal routines and a refreshing night's sleep.

Daylight saving

Daylight saving is a boon to adults and a curse to parents. While the parents may enjoy the extra hours of the evening available for leisure, they are concerned about bedtimes. Regular bedtime is important as an anchor point for estab-lishing night-time sleep.

Every year I see frustrated families who have spent weeks

arranging a good night's sleep with their child waking at about 6.30 a.m. Daylight saving arrives, and then 6.30 is suddenly 5.30 a.m.

Most often I encourage my patients to have their baby in bed to start the night between 6.30 and 7.30, preferably the former. Once this has been achieved and the child is sleeping for 10 to 12 hours, life improves, and the parents feel a greater sense of control.

What happens, though, when suddenly the nation ignores the 6.30 bedtime you have so carefully established with your baby, and now calls that time 5.30 or 7.30? This sudden change to the clock can disrupt your ability to manage bedtime.

It is common for parents to come back to me a month after the start of daylight saving because they have 'lost it'. After weeks of working on a program that suited mother, father and child, they are now back where they started.

The problem seems to be caused not by the change in time, but by the family's response to it. Many parents attempt to accommodate the change in time by trying to maintain the bedtime relative to the sun. Bedtime may have been, for instance, 7 p.m. before daylight saving commenced, so to continue 'as before', the child is put down at 8 p.m. according to the clock. This is sensible, rational, understandable, and wrong.

The problem is that, in all other areas, family life quickly adjusts to the clock and is not ruled by the sun. The baby adjusts to the changed family routine, moves his waking time to coincide with the rest of the family, but is going to bed at 8 p.m. and not 7 p.m. He thus loses an hour or part of an hour's sleep per night. He becomes a little more tired, and this begins to interfere with his sleep skills. The program of sleep begins to unravel, with nights becoming difficult again. This is sad after so much hard work.

Because the entry point to the problem was a logical decision, it is difficult to see the way forward. So how do we avoid the problem?

Because life in our culture is time orientated, and not so clearly sun orientated, we need to work *by the clock*.

The problem here is that 7 p.m. on Saturday suddenly becomes 8 p.m. on Sunday. How do we put the child down an hour 'earlier'? The answer is to move bedtime back a few minutes each day. Thus, if we assume 7 p.m. Saturday is converted to 8 p.m. Sunday, the bedtimes I would recommend are as follows:

Sunday	7.45 p.m.
Monday	7.30 p.m.
Tuesday	7.15 p.m.
Wednesday	7.00 p.m.

This then returns all members of the family to a position that works both in terms of organising the day and achieving the required amount of sleep for the baby.

This strategy should work for the majority of families, and you can enjoy the advantages. Once the baby has returned to normal sleep times, you have an extra hour of sunshine on a summer evening to work or relax as you see fit. A glass of wine with your partner is recommended while you both enjoy the peaceful silence as the sun sets.

Illness

Illness is almost inevitable for children at some time.

There are different rules of management when a baby is unwell with a high temperature or vomiting, diarrhoea, etc. It is inappropriate to leave such a child alone throughout the night. There will be a need to monitor the temperature, check on nappies and bedding, and observe general well-being. The problem is the effect this will have on the child's sleep patterns when she has recovered normal health.

As I have repeated many times in this book, sleep achievement is in part cue dependent. Cues of sleep are learned. Parents are very powerful reward structures and will rapidly be incorporated into a style of sleep achievement. Even the sick child monitors her environment and has the ability to re-learn cues of sleep. Thus, as one or other parent has been coming in two or three times a night to check on the child during the episode of ill health, this rapidly becomes the preferred option once the illness is over. The parents are aware that their baby is well again, but they are being 'politely' requested to attend and provide a little comfort once or twice throughout the night. This is particularly frustrating for a family that has struggled to achieve good sleep routines. It is discouraging to have good sleep routines destroyed by a cold which has lasted only three or four days.

There is an answer. The child is behaving logically. She has indicated a preference for parental contact and this preference is strong enough for her to wake fully and cry out. The parents' response needs to contain two elements. First, you need to understand that the child is behaving normally and is not being naughty or difficult. Second, you know that before the illness your child had a proven ability to sleep throughout the night. It is now time to gently but firmly insist that the child return to those patterns.

You can tackle this in either of two ways. The gentle approach is to attend at the child's cry during the night, but gradually decreasing the time you spend with her over two, three or four nights. Make it less and less rewarding for her to expend energy on calling for you overnight. The tougher approach is to not re-attend during the night in response to a call. As long as you are sure that the child is well and safe, do nothing. Once you are confident that the child is asleep then you may feel better if you go in to check that all is well and to replace the covering over your baby if it has been dislodged during active sleep or by the effort of calling for your company.

The first approach is slower, but kinder to your emotions. It can be traumatic to leave a child to cry herself to sleep when she is recovering from a recent illness. The second approach is faster, but requires commitment from the parents.

'Losing it' following an episode of illness is very common. I hope the above strategy helps get things back on track.

Moving house or moving interstate

Moving is common in our mobile society. Unfortunately it is also a common cause of losing control of a carefully established sleep routine.

There are two elements to the loss of control: different cues of sleep, and fatigue. I discuss fatigue in the next section when I address moving overseas. The main problem in moving house is the different cues of sleep.

When you move into a new house, flat or caravan there are, of course, many changes. In the new home, there are changes in the cues of sleep. There are different colours, room sizes and, in particular, different background noises. One family I saw lived on a boat, and it was very hard on their baby when they came to live on land. For the first time ever, the 'home' did not rock and sway all night! Most adults are able to relate to the effect of different sounds at night interfering with sleep. Once you understand the role that cues of sleep play, then it is logical to see that the child may lose the routine while new and different cues are being learned.

Sleep achievement is facilitated by a complex group of factors, including tiredness and cues. The child will be tired in the evening, which works to your advantage. You already understand the importance of avoiding overtiredness. What I would like to emphasise here is that there are also some cues which you carry with you, and which work to your advantage. There are many things which you can do in the same way at your new home which will be familiar to the infant, and so will assist in sleep achievement.

Time

Keep bedtime about the same.

Routine

The things you would normally do should be repeated to the best of your ability.

Patience

The child may take longer to achieve sleep, so do not feel threatened. Use the program of minimal reassurance and within a few days the child's sleep skills will return to normal.

While I know that this all sounds idealised, particularly when the house is topsy-turvy, and you can't find the baby bath let alone keep bedtime to a regular 7 p.m., it does work. The most optimistic statement I can make is that once the child has gone to sleep, it leaves you free to get on with the other vital tasks, like finding that box labelled 'kitchen' containing tomorrow's breakfast.

Moving overseas

By moving overseas I am really talking about travelling long distances, such as to the USA or Europe. If the family is moving a shorter distance, from Sydney to New Zealand, say, the advice is the same as for moving house and adjusting to daylight saving. Moving overseas is a challenge. Holidaying overseas with a child is twice the challenge because you not only go away, you then come back. The baby's sleep routines are disrupted at least twice.

With long-distance overseas travel, two factors are added to the usual problems of moving. These are fatigue and body or 'circadian' rhythms.

Fatigue

Fatigue and overtiredness are powerful factors interfering with sleep achievement. Most of you will have experienced the joys of trying to settle a child who is severely overtired and has totally lost the plot. With long journeys, such as 24 hours in a plane, there is no routine. The time of day constantly changes, and depending upon your direction of travel you may even lose or gain a whole day.

For the infant, the enemy here is tiredness. There is no easy solution apart from being aware. Every hour of sleep that can be achieved for the baby or child will help. If you have a chance anywhere, at any time, to help the child sleep for an hour or two, then use it. It is most unlikely that the child will achieve normal hours of sleep while travelling, but do your best.

This is one setting where I find that antihistamine sedatives have a place. See your general practitioner and get advice on sedation for your child—and possibly yourself. If a little antihistamine improves sleep on the journey, it may help avoid the problems of fatigue.

Circadian rhythms

Once you reach your destination, there are two significant problems for infant sleep. The child is now tired or overtired because of disrupted sleep on the plane, and because the body clock or circadian rhythms are out of alignment by twelve hours or thereabouts.

You may be aware that there is a gland in the brain which secretes a sleep-inducing chemical called melatonin in response to day and night, that is to light and dark cycles. This gland is cycling for, say, Australia, but you are now in London. It is understandable that there will be difficulty in establishing night sleep when the child's body is expecting daytime activities.

The best advice is to apply your old routines as soon as possible. Adjust your activities to the clock of your new destination, keep night-time as dark as is practicable, and if the child wants a happy wake time at 2 a.m., be reluctant to participate to the best of your ability.

During the day, use every opportunity to achieve sleep for both yourself and the child. Every hour of sleep during the day is a contribution towards the recovery of a normal sleep cycle. The exception here is if a young child, say six months old, tries to sleep for six or more hours straight during the day. In this case there may be problems at night. Set a daytime limit of approximately four to five hours, and then wake the child for feeding. If he is still tired after the feed, allow him to return to sleep.

It will take several days for the body's biology to adjust to the new location, but it does happen.

Two keys here, then, are to avoid overtiredness to the best of your ability, and to apply your old routines at the local times as soon as possible.

When you return from overseas, all of the above applies again.

Bon voyage!

Visitors

The final cause of 'losing it' I will discuss is visitors.

For the family, visits from aunts, uncles and grandparents can be exciting but disruptive events. Some homes are large enough to accommodate the relative with routines unchanged. (If this is the case, read no further.) For many families, though, a visiting friend or relative requires a change in routine and possibly a change in bedroom for the child or baby.

If this applies to you, here are a couple of strategies to follow.

Resist overhandling, prolonged playtimes and delays in bedtime because your child is spending time with the loved relative. This may require some diplomatic skills, particularly if Nanna or Grandpa has come a long way and just wants to 'help you' by nursing the baby for a considerable time. Explain your need for routine to maintain good quality sleep. To the best of your ability make the visitor an ally in the sleep program.

Unfortunately, some relatives are so overwhelming in their loving that all you can do is count down the days. To the best of your ability, prevent overtiredness and overhandling. Of course, on the other hand, it may be wonderful to have an extra person to help you during the day.

Another problem may be caused by the child sleeping in

a different room. This is particularly so if it is your room, and this is not what you are used to. The noises of a sleeping baby or child and their little cries may be disruptive to you or your partner. Conversely, if the child is old enough to recognise that her parents are more available, she may want to come into bed 'for just a minute'.

Problems can be compounded by not wanting to allow a child to cry through the night and disturb the visitor. Stick to your overnight routine to the best of your ability. Explain to the visitor that there may be some overnight noise. Many conflicts can be avoided by explaining the situation. If your visitor becomes an ally, life becomes easier.

Once the visitor leaves, return to your normal routine.

Failure

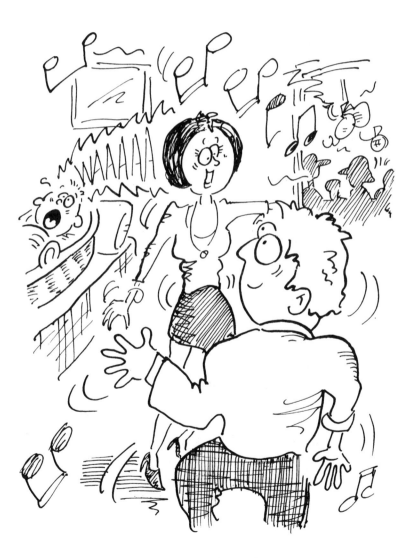

IT IS WITH DEEP REGRET that I announce that my advice is
not universally successful. Over the years I have used these
failures as an opportunity to observe and learn why they
occur. This chapter attempts to explain the common causes
of failure to achieve acceptable sleep patterns.

Parents of young children are under immense pressure
from both their personal expectations and those of their
family and friends. Our society places a high value on
parenting, and as it is one of our major endeavours in life
we try hard to do it very well. This high expectation is accompanied by the realities of tiredness and often little experience.
When a new parent confronts a baby who is crying for what
seems to be hours and hours, things sometimes go wrong.

I am very much aware that the parents who come to see
me for their first visit have often received advice from people
from different organisations and of different philosophies.
Occasionally the parents will report to me that they have just
come from a respected organisation which has given them
exactly the opposite advice. Parents are often left with the
unenviable task of making a choice between opposing points
of view. I am not in the least surprised when the people I
am seeing, after having thought through the information
I give them, choose another philosophy for the care of their
children. In fact, I am regularly impressed and grateful for
the high proportion of parents who are willing to give my
ideas at least a try.

Despite this there are still failures, and I have been encouraged to document the common causes of failure in achieving
good control of infant sleep. I will discuss these under a
number of broad headings.

In general the causes include the following, in no particular order:

- lack of spouse support

- an inconsistent approach
- genuine ill health
- hunger
- sabotage
- an incompatible philosophy
- difficult children
- lifestyle.

In any given family there may be one or a combination of two or more of the above factors.

Lack of spouse support

A majority of infants will spend time crying when learning independent sleep skills. It is distressing and tiring for a parent to do nothing while an infant is crying himself to sleep. I know from my own experience as a father that, at two o'clock in the morning, doing nothing while your baby is crying is much harder than doing something. It takes a considerable commitment from parents. To a certain extent, in the initial days of the program, before improvement occurs, it is an act of faith to do nothing. This time spent doing nothing is not restful for you, the parent. It may be that one of the parents is less convinced than the other and will not support the idea of waiting until sleep is achieved. A variation on this theme is the partner who makes the comment 'I have got to work in the morning. I need my sleep. Get up and do something about the baby!'

These points of view are entirely understandable. However, they do put the more committed parent in a difficult position. Sometimes this pressure will be so significant that the parent is unable to continue to ignore the infant's crying and is forced to attend to the child. The result is that the pattern of developing sleep skills is lost. Unfortunately this turns a short-term problem into a long-term problem. The sleep problem which may have been controlled in one to two weeks is now converted into a trend which continues to occur for months, and, in some unfortunate cases, for years.

There is no magic solution to the problem of inadequate support from one's partner. In consulting, I attempt to get both parents to the first consultation. If I explain the philosophy to both it is far more likely that they will support each other.

Parenting is a challenging job, particularly when you are learning new skills while being tired. It is made doubly difficult if your partner fails to support you. This text may prove useful in obtaining help from your companion.

Inconsistent approach

Inconsistency is probably the dominant cause of failure. The sequence of events is relatively easy to explain. Families that come to see me are often trying multiple methods recommended by several advisers. Everyone has an opinion; everyone has advice. As the method used by the family varies from day to day, little may be achieved.

The underlying philosophy of the book is that we are teaching the child the skill of achieving sleep independently. When teaching any skill, be it the alphabet or tables, how to throw a ball or to sleep successfully, a consistent approach usually produces the best outcome.

The dangers of inconsistency are twofold. In the first place, many methods are being tried and no method is taken to a successful conclusion. The second danger is more profound and can have negative effects in the long term. This second area of inconsistency works as follows.

Let us assume that the family has decided to try the method outlined in this book. The child is well, gaining weight, and no problem can be identified that could cause wakefulness. When the baby is fed, bathed, and prepared for bed, she is left on her own for gradually increasing periods of time. The child is reassured for short periods of time by a gentle touch, gentle rearrangement in the bed or cot or bassinet, and a few affectionate words. She is then left to settle off to sleep alone. Contact time might be 30 to 90 seconds, and separation may be 5, 10, 15, 20 minutes or more. Let us also assume that the child is being taught to sleep independently, as opposed to achieving sleep in her mother's or father's arms and then sleeping for large parts of the night in the parental bed.

On the first night the parents are determined, and they eventually find that the child achieves sleep, but only after a considerable amount of crying. On the second night they are again determined, and although the crying is less, it still disturbs their sleep. On the third night, all is quiet until 2 a.m. Then the baby awakens with a loud cry. After 30 minutes, one partner has had enough, and says, 'Look I know what we should be doing, but I'm tired. I've got to work early tomorrow. Let's bring the baby into bed, get a decent sleep, and start again tomorrow.' The trap here, in what is a very understandable scenario, is that we have given mixed messages to the infant. For two nights, the reward of parental company was stopped or minimised. On the third night the reward of parental company is given for the behaviour pattern of crying for attention. This intermittent or irregular reward is like an occasional win on a poker machine. It is a powerful training tool for the behaviour pattern of continuing to cry. The baby has thus been rewarded for crying for two nights. Crying has now become useful behaviour. As we now have a baby who has been rewarded for persistent crying, the problem is worse than when it started.

The moral of the story is that once the family has decided to use parent-independent cues of sleep, and once you have decided to help the child learn to achieve sleep alone, you need to continue until you are successful.

Not everyone has the determination or the family circumstances to allow this. My pointing out this pitfall may help you to avoid it.

Ill health

One of the assumptions of this book is that your child is in good health. Not all children are well. There are children who suffer genuine painful reflux, pyloric stenosis, urinary infections, asthma, pneumonia, severe prematurity, or a host of other serious conditions. A short-term illness should be just a minor disruption (page 148), but long-term ill health can make the teaching of sleep skills difficult, impossible, or inappropriate.

It is difficult to give guidelines about ill health and sleep disorders. Each case has to be treated on its merits. The most useful general comment is that when the child is struggling with ill health, good sleep is to everyone's advantage. If it is not dangerous to the child to teach independent sleep skills, then try to achieve good quality sleep as soon as practical.

If the ill health continues for years, a solution to the sleeping problems will eventually need to be found. For example, one of my three-year-old patients was born with a disease that is normally fatal. The child's life expectancy was six months. Quite clearly, in this setting, sleep was not a priority. Through one of life's miracles, the disease did not proceed to damage the child. By age three, she was bright, capable, healthy (considering her disease), and completely in control of the family. Bedtime, according to the young lady, was between midnight and one a.m., and then only if she was held in her mother's arms. The family was exhausted. I did find a solution for this family, but the focus of this section is health problems. I am telling this story here as an interesting paradox. I am not suggesting that illness should be ignored. If your child is experiencing genuine ill health then that should be given priority over teaching sleep skills.

Hunger

Hunger is a possible cause of sleeplessness and crying, and needs to be addressed before you attempt to teach sleep skills. It is understandable for a child to wake up and demand attention when he is genuinely hungry. This is possibly the second most common cause of sleep problems, particularly in the first three months. The hungry baby will understandably resist any attempts at training to achieve prolonged sleep.

Checking hunger as a cause of sleeplessness can be difficult when you are breast feeding. The easiest technique is to check weight gain. (See page 10.) If the baby is growing at a rate of 30 gram per day or better during the first three months, then hunger is probably not the cause of sleeplessness. Having said that I must add that some infants do achieve very rapid growth, and the occasional infant, often male, can gain weight at a rate of 50 to 60 gram per day.

Advice on supporting successful breast feeding is given in Chapter 1.

Parents who are bottle feeding usually have less cause for concern about hunger as the volume taken is so easily observed.

Sabotage

This is a tricky area.

The parents have decided that they wish to pursue a particular style of sleep for their family. Sometimes this includes an amount of 'crying down'. Other relatives may not approve and this may be shown in different ways. It may present as direct opposition: 'How can you let my grand-daughter cry. It's not healthy. She will develop a hernia. Let me pick her up. See, she's quiet in my arms. This is your first baby. I'll show you how. I will rock her to sleep.'

There are two problems here. The first is that relatives go home and leave you with the problems they cause. The second is that the child is once again receiving mixed messages about cues of sleep and this interferes with the learning process.

The second type of sabotage may be more subtle. Some-times a relative shares the care of a child. For example, a grandparent may look after the child on a regular basis, perhaps for a couple of nights a week or during the day, because the child's parents work. The time when the grand-parent (or any other carer) is sharing care can be used by them as a time to use a different style of sleep achievement. This may be constructive or destructive.

There is only one solution, and that is to explain the program to your relatives or other carer in as much detail as you need to obtain their support. Consistency is very important to the process of learning.

Occasionally grandparents send messages of protest to me via the family I am seeing. 'This baby sleeps too much.' 'When can I get a chance to hold my grandchild?' The answer to such an inquiry/protest is that the child will be a member of the family for a long time. Please let us establish good feeding, sleeping, and growth. The child will grow quickly and within a few months there will be ample time for playing and all the other joys of being an active grandparent.

Incompatible philosophy

The underlying philosophy of this book is that good quality sleep promotes happy interaction between family members. Sleep achievement is in part a learned skill. Sometimes a child must be left alone and given the chance to achieve sleep independently or with only a little parental input and reassurance. This may include some 'crying down' to sleep.

Some parents do not share this philosophy. It is argued by some authorities that, particularly in the first six months of life, the baby's cry is a signal representing a genuine need. They may add that to ignore the cry is harmful to the child's psychological well-being.

Working with children has taught me that the above analysis is incomplete and can lead to unsuccessful approaches to sleep routines. It is a philosophy which fails to recognise the role of fatigue, in my experience the dominant cause of infant crying. If the cause of the crying is tiredness, then the solution is sleep. Endless hours of rocking or patting or feeding or driving around the block may provide periods of quiet, but they do not provide the good quality sleep that is required. In fact, all this handling may keep the child awake, decrease the amount of sleep achieved, increase the level of tiredness, and thus worsen the problem.

Another element of the philosophy mentioned above is often that the more physical contact between child and parent, the better. One reference suggests that if you want to be a serious mother you should hold your baby 24 hours per day for the first five years.

My answer is as follows. Parenting is wonderful. It should be fulfilling, engaging and pleasurable. It is difficult to feel pleasure, to enjoy any relationship with any member of the family, or even think logically, if your brain is numbed by fatigue. Sleeping times are for sleep, feeding times are for feeding, and play times are for play. When it is time for a child to sleep, let the child sleep. Let the parents have some time for each other and then enjoy a full night's sleep. They can then wake in the morning looking forward to spending the day with their child.

If your philosophy is incompatible with this book, then my advice will be irrelevant. You have probably given up before reading far. Let's hope that your children belong to that 70 per cent of children who sleep well anyway.

Difficult children

Some children have medical problems that interfere with mental development. Mental retardation, brain injury, and autism are just a few examples. This is a complex area, and the family involved will require specialist advice. This book assumes that you are dealing with normal healthy children.

The sleep literature discusses children with difficult 'temperaments'. The argument goes that children with difficult temperaments may sleep poorly. Which comes first though, the difficult temperament causing poor sleep, or poor sleep resulting in an understandably negative temperament?

The policy I use is that almost all children have a pleasant temperament once they have adequate food, sleep and love. As with all philosophies, life will occasionally choose not to agree. It seems to work almost all of the time. I hope your children fit the pattern.

Having said this, I acknowledge that there are children who may be extremely testing. As early as approximately six months of age, some children appear to be able to hold a clear image of what they wish to achieve. Their parents may report that they know it has become a battle of wills. Some parents even tell me that they are aware of having lost the battle. They are sure that the child or baby is in control.

My advice is to take control. Almost always, you do know best about what is correct and in the baby's best interest. Over the years I have observed some heroic battles between parents and children. One of the ironies in this situation is that the child who wins about food or sleep almost always makes a bad choice. For example, he may behave in a way that results in limited sleep. He is then overtired and unhappy. The children who are led by their parents to constructive and appropriate feeding and sleeping patterns tend to be happier.

Lifestyle

Have you ever heard someone say at a social gathering, 'We're expecting our first child. We're really excited but we're planning to continue our present lifestyle. The baby will have to fit in with us.' Those of you who already have children may smile reassuringly and think, 'They've got a shock coming.'

The reality is that children bring a major change in lifestyle for almost all of us. Our personal needs, wants and desires take a back seat to caring for a wonderful new human who is totally reliant upon us, and who doesn't happen to know the meaning of the words, 'Please be reasonable, I need some time out right now.'

Most families make the necessary adjustments to their lifestyle, and enjoy the pleasures of parenting. Some, however, continue to have irregular meal times and bedtimes, and a general absence of daytime routines. This does not work to the advantage of young children developing feeding and sleeping patterns. It can, however, be an insoluble problem if this is the established pattern for the family. These lifestyle problems tend to continue through the different generations of a family.

Conclusion

Not everyone will be successful in achieving good sleep patterns for their children. The causes of failure are multiple. The most common are tiredness (of the infant), hunger, and an inconsistent approach by the parents. Other problems with partners and relatives also occur. The relevant sections above should give you some useful guidance.

Colic and other issues

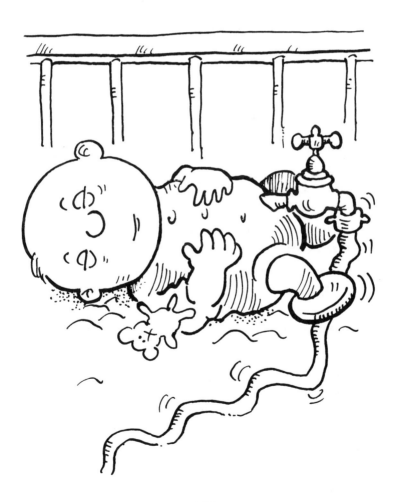

THIS CHAPTER IS A collection of pieces of advice which may be useful but which do not fit logically in a chapter on their own or with other pieces of information.

Colic

Colic is mentioned several times in this book. It is a very common diagnosis in circles discussing child care. Colic exists. It can be very troublesome and cause significant anxiety and sleeplessness. Unfortunately, I think that it is a diagnosis that is overused and often applied incorrectly. In my own practice I regard colic as a diagnosis of exclusion, or, to put it another way, it is my last choice as a diagnosis.

For many parents, 'colic' simply means that the baby is crying. The most common causes of the baby's crying are hunger and overtiredness. These need to be excluded first. The hungry baby will respond to being fed; end of problem. The overtired baby is discussed extensively elsewhere in this book. Overtiredness needs to be excluded as well as hunger before retreating to the diagnosis of colic.

The cause of colic is not known as far as I am aware. The child suffering from colic is otherwise well and for most of the day behaves well. Typically the child is well fed, lying in a clean dry nappy, and should be going to sleep. Unfortunately she is tearful and difficult to settle. The time tends to be late in the day, although this is not universal. If she is examined by a doctor, generally nothing untoward is found.

Fortunately the majority of babies grow out of colic by twelve weeks of age. What, however, do we do while we are waiting for the problem to go away?

Treatment tends to have limited success. Be sure in your own mind that the baby has had sufficient to drink, check that the nappy is clean and dry, and make sure that the wraps are firm while at the same time the baby is not over-wrapped and hot. Some paracetamol may be helpful; if nothing else it helps the parents to know that they have done something. Once these steps have been taken it may be necessary to stand back and wait for the baby to settle. This can be hard.

The baby with colic looks and sounds very unhappy. She cries very loudly. Tears may run down her cheeks. She may pull up her legs as if in pain. Generally she is difficult to console and does not want to feed. Fortunately, once you have waited the 15 or 30 or 60 minutes that the baby takes to settle, she does sleep successfully, and then she wakes cheerfully as if there had never been a problem. Your thoughts may be a little ungenerous next morning after the beaming child has had you up several times overnight.

There are no hard and fast rules on what can cause colic, and different babies behave differently. However, riding in the pusher on a windy day and driving in the car can increase episodes which we may call colic. Driving in the car is interesting. Most parents find that children travel well in the car; perhaps the noise and movement is reassuring. The problem arises *after* the journey. That night may be more difficult with the child being tearful and unsettled.

Treatment is the same as for overtired babies. Once the child is well fed, clean and appropriately wrapped, put her down and leave her alone to achieve sleep. Again I repeat that this can be difficult and stressful for the parents, particularly when she is your first child. But forewarned is forearmed.

Nappy rash

This topic is included here for two reasons. First, one of my friends who used the original version of the book asked me to write about the topic, as she had problems with her child. Second, like so many things that can go wrong with a young child, nappy rash can be severe enough to make parents worry that it may be causing sleeplessness. So this is my short effort at giving advice on nappy area care.

I do not propose to enter the debate about whether disposable nappies are good or bad from society's viewpoint. The reality is that large numbers of babies are wearing large numbers of disposable nappies. My comments below really relate to cloth nappies because disposable nappies are more efficient at removing moisture from contact with the skin. If using disposables, you can approximately halve the recommended rate of nappy changes. Thus, while I generally recommend twelve cloth nappies per day, six disposables is probably adequate on an average day when the baby's skin is healthy.

Nappy rash is one of the most common problems seen by the general practitioner. Sometimes the nappy area is infected with thrush or affected by dermatitis. In the majority of cases, the skin in the nappy area is suffering from moisture damage.

A baby passes small volumes of urine frequently, perhaps as often as every fifteen minutes. What this means is that if the nappy is changed hourly, i.e. 24 times per day, then the nappy area would be wet for 18 hours a day. If any adult left their hands in water for 18 hours a day the skin would become red and cracked. It is little wonder that babies get nappy rash. Perhaps the question should be why all babies don't get it more severely than they do.

Some hints on nappy area care, but please note that these comments relate to cloth nappies. Change as often as possible: before and after feeds possibly, between feeds if the baby has been disturbed for some reason. Perhaps change as you are going to bed. Definitely change as soon as possible after a bowel action as it can burn the skin. Aim to use a minimum of 12 nappies per day.

Despite the most intense care, some babies will still get a degree of nappy rash.

Nappy rash is the response of the skin to moisture and the chemicals in that moisture, that is to urine and the waste products in that urine. If the skin can be protected from the moisture then it is less prone to break down. A water repellent layer of petroleum jelly (Vaseline), lanolin, zinc cream, or one of many other products may be helpful.

Obviously, the more often these protective layers are applied the better. Washing the nappy in a pure soap such as Lux or Velvet instead of a detergent washing powder will also be of benefit. In addition, make certain that the nappies are well rinsed.

If, despite your best efforts, the child still develops nappy rash, see the doctor.

Toilet training

This is not an area for which I claim great experience as it tends not to be the focus of my consulting. Despite this, it is raised often enough for me to offer some advice.

Luckily, the problem of toilet training is nowhere as intrusive as sleep disturbance. Children almost always develop control of bladder or bowel with a little encouragement, while sleep disturbance may persist for years unless a solution is found.

With many children we seem to delay toilet training longer than necessary. Some of the experienced parents who have spoken to me suspect that if training is started later in life the child is more likely to object and delay success.

Some children are capable of achieving bladder and bowel control earlier than others. One point which needs to be remembered about toilet training is the need for consistency. Do not start if you know that for some reason there will be a change of pattern after a few days. For example, it is ineffective to begin training if you are going on holidays a few days after starting. The problem is that this gives inconsistent signals to the infant. Just as it is important to give consistent signals in teaching sleep skills, so in teaching toileting skills be consistent and persistent. And as with sleep skills, other care givers need to apply the same approach.

Bowel

Early bowel training requires three elements to be successful. The child needs to be able to sit up, to have reasonably regular bowel habits or at least indicate clearly to you that he is starting to use his bowel, and finally you need to want to try.

Once the child can sit up, and you know or strongly suspect that a bowel movement is about to occur, reach for the potty. Sit the child on the pot and allow him to complete the bowel action there. If nothing happens, that's fine. If the child does empty his bowel in the pot, then you should 'congratulate' him. The more often such a successful event occurs, the more rapidly the child develops this as a habit. Because it happens in your company, it is also safe and secure. Eventually he starts to pass urine at the same time.

How early can you begin? This is entirely up to you. Some

mothers have started as early as six months, although that is unusual. Most children should be able to start by twelve months. Success is not instantaneous; training will take weeks or months.

Bladder

In the area of bladder training I assume that a dry bottom is more comfortable than a wet one.

At a time that you decide is appropriate, take the child out of nappies during the day. In preparation for this you will need lots of pairs of underpants. At every passing of urine in the pants, change the pants as soon as you notice. Encourage passing of urine in the toilet or on the pot. Make it a winning game as much as possible. Passing urine on the toilet should be rewarded with congratulations, kisses, hugs, etc. Wet pants result in a change of pants. Note that the rewards here are only positive. After some time the child may recognise that dry bottoms are more comfortable, and begin to seek out the pot or the toilet.

Night-time dryness is related to the bladder's ability to accept a larger volume of urine before emptying by reflex. The mistake to make is that of encouraging frequent empty-ing. This results in a lower holding volume for the bladder and worsening of night-time wetting. Of course, family his-tory is important, and if either parent developed night-time bladder control late in life, the children may also be late.

ADD/ADHD

Attention deficit disorder and attention deficit hyperactivity disorder are common problems. Between 1 to 4 per cent of children are affected, and 80 per cent of affected children are boys.

The reason for raising the diagnosis in this book is twofold. The first is to note that sleep disorders are frequently noted in children with one or other of these problems. The second is that my personal, presently unpublished research shows that sleep problems may have been present from an early age. These studies using retrospective surveys showed poor sleep performance as early as three months.

I make no claims whatsoever as to whether sleep deprivation causes ADHD or if they are both elements of one syndrome, or even that fatigue unmasks ADHD. It is simply clear that sleep problems are common in these children. It is difficult to conceive that assisting the child to achieve good sleep as early as possible in life could be harmful. It is impossible to say if better sleep skills will protect against ADHD, avoid it emerging as a problem, or have no effect at all. However, I repeat that it can do no harm to you, your child or your family to develop good sleep skills early in life. At the very least we do know that better sleep leads to improved family functioning.

Teething

Teething causes much debate. The presence of, absence of, and movement of teeth is blamed for everything from sleepless nights to changes in almost every bodily function up to and including nappy rash.

It is very difficult to ask a baby of six months if her teeth are hurting. Certainly as we grow into that part of our life for which we retain memory, teething is painless. I know about wisdom teeth, but that is a different problem caused by crowding, not the eruption of teeth.

I well remember a prominent British paediatrician speaking to me when I was a medical student and saying with great authority: 'Teething produces teeth and nothing else.' At the time, I thought he was an old fuddy-duddy who had probably never personally cared for a baby 24 hours a day in his life. I have come full circle, and I think he was right. (Have I become the fuddy-duddy?)

Over the years, many parents have come to me concerned that their child's sleep problems are caused by teething. I have the greatest success when ignoring teething as a problem.

Occasionally, despite my reassurance, the parents are convinced that teething is the problem. In this setting I recommend regular paracetamol overnight, say every four to six hours as indicated by the child's distress. The parents are then reassured that their child has received appropriate care for what they, the parents, believe is a painful condition. Taken as directed, paracetamol is very safe, and the parents feel more comfortable.

As a rule, I recommend that you adopt the following attitudes:
- Teething produces teeth.
- Teething is a normal process.
- If the baby is unsettled, teething is probably not the cause.

If you adopt the above beliefs, you will almost always be correct.

The danger in believing in painful teething is to be seduced into providing lots of reassuring cuddles, walks around the house etc. based upon the belief that the child is distressed. The consequence can be that the child rapidly adopts parent-dependent cues for sleep transitions, and then disrupted sleep becomes the norm.

Having said all that, I will write in the escape clause. Over the years I have certainly seen children who had recurring colds and ear infections, which were painful, and which appeared to come very close to the time of the appearance of new teeth.

Sedatives

Sedation with drugs such as Vallergan, Progan or other anti-histamines is often recommended to families with a child who is sleeping poorly.

I rarely use drugs in the care of sleepless children. The reason for this is that it does not help in the long term.

Let me return to my basic points. Sleep achievement is a learned skill. If sleep is generated by a chemical then the child's learning processes are not involved. I can put anyone to sleep with an anaesthetic. Using these chemicals or drugs does not help the person receiving them learn anything. Once the chemicals are withdrawn the family is back where it began.

There are exceptions. Antihistamine sedatives can be useful, and I feel comfortable with parents planning to use them when they are undertaking prolonged travel. If you are going to be driving or flying for a day or two, there will be many opportunities for your baby to miss sleep. A sedative-induced sleep can be useful in guarding against overtiredness when you reach your destination.

Another occasion in which I recommend sedation is the severely stressed family. If the parents feel that they are not coping because of severe exhaustion then any sleep can be important. The objective for the family in this setting is survival, not perfection. Sedating the infant and possibly the parents for a few nights may be essential before beginning training in sleep skills.

In conclusion, the following is useful to remember:

- Sedatives are rarely useful in the long term.
- Sedative-induced sleep does not usually lead to improved sleep performance by children once the drug is stopped.
- If the family is suffering severely from sleep deprivation then short-term use may be valuable in providing a rest for the parents.
- When travelling for long periods, there may be a place for some sedation to help avoid overtiredness.
- Obtain advice on what drugs and what dosage to use from an appropriately trained health-care professional.

Sex and parenthood

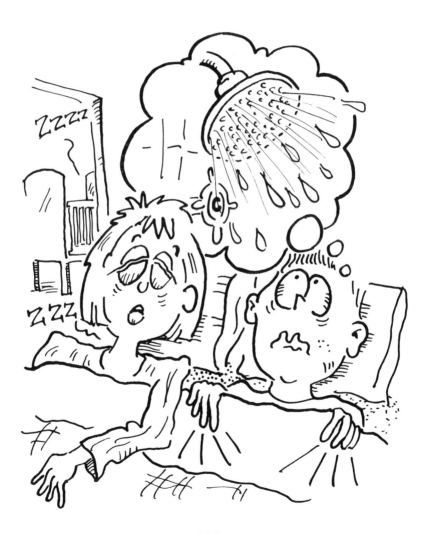

LIFE IS FULL OF contradictions. For example, there is no parenthood without sex. Once parenthood is achieved, however, it does not mean an uninterrupted sexual coexistence. Sexuality is one of the casualties of parenthood. Having achieved its desired aim or perhaps, more accurately, one of its aims, sexuality becomes a victim of its own success.

If you are among those parents who have an uninterrupted sexual relationship after the birth of their children, congratulations, read no further. If you are among those who have experienced the occasional problem, read on. You are not alone.

If you find that parenthood has led to a significant decrease in the frequency and enthusiasm for making love, there are explanations. There is also some good news: it will return. *Eventually.*

Men are interesting creatures. They are fairly predictable. The majority have a continuing interest in making love despite the ups and downs of life. Very few say no if sex is offered. Most are perplexed when sex is not offered 'like before'. The sometimes dramatic change in sexual activity after the birth of a child can be threatening to a man's perception of himself.

Making love is an important expression of mutual affection and attraction. In our society most men place great emphasis upon making love successfully and frequently. When, after the birth of a child, the woman is suddenly very much less interested, it is easy to see this as a loss of interest or affection. In fact the causes are much more complex. Sexuality is hormone-dependent to a very significant extent. A man who loses his testes and thus his testosterone has no sexual drive. Most men, however, retain their testes and produce testosterone in adequate and fairly constant volumes. Their interest in sexuality is thus fairly constant.

A woman is also strongly influenced by the hormones in circulation in her body. Most women would agree that there are days of the month when their partners are attractive and when love-making is pleasant. Conversely, there are days of the month when their partners are attractive but love-making is not on the agenda. The exact time of the month varies, but most women are most receptive around ovulation. The reproductive sense of this is obvious.

While a woman is breast feeding there is usually an inhibition of ovulation and the hormonal variations that go with it. As the woman's interest may peak around ovulation, if she is not ovulating there may be little interest.

Once a child is born two important things happen. First, the woman's hormones undergo a major change, and second, she is doing a huge amount of work. The baby who is breast fed and getting pleasantly round is getting all of that energy for growth from his mother. The mother is putting out that energy from her body. In addition to that there is the physical work of caring for house, children, clothing, partner, shopping, work etc. So, men, if your partner says she is too tired tonight, what she probably means is 'I'm exhausted. It's difficult to do another solitary thing without some sleep.'

Is there any good news here?

Well, an end is in sight. Breast feeding will finish eventually. As the months go by the baby should come into a routine that allows the mother more rest, and this frees up energy for other things.

There is a most important point about a man's masculinity and attractiveness. In the woman's eyes he is just as manly and attractive. It is just that circumstances beyond her control do not allow her to express it as frequently or with the same enthusiasm as before the pregnancy and birth of the child.

It is tragic to see a couple being torn apart through a lack of understanding of these issues. The man must be allowed to realise that the absence of sexual activity is not a comment upon his masculinity. The woman deserves understanding and support at a time when her body is working extremely hard.

A major reward for the partner who is understanding and supportive is that, as time goes by, his actions strengthen the relationship. When his companion's energy returns she will have more regard and love for him. The sexuality of this maturing relationship may be more meaningful and satisfying in the long term.

Patient comment

Dear Dr Symon,

I am writing to you in appreciation for all that you have done for my son Matthew and our marriage.

My husband and I were in such a dilemma with Matthew who was constantly crying day and night with no sleep pattern. It did not seem to matter whatever we did for him; we were unable to settle Matthew. We visited numerous general practitioners, doctors at the children's hospital, and specialists to no avail. Matthew went through all the formulas on the market and different colic medication; the medical profession blamed his sleep disorder on colic. The only compensation they gave was that he would grow out of it. In the meanwhile, with sleepless nights, my husband and I were not coping. It started affecting our marriage. We hired a nurse and family help to give us some relief. Financially we were not able to continue.

We heard of your service on childhood sleep disorders through my husband's friends. Seeing that we had exhausted all other avenues and for our own sanity, we decided to try it. We were amazed and astonished that since therapy

Matthew is put to bed at 6.30 p.m. sharp and doesn't wake until 6.30 a.m. Matthew is a very active child with a mind of his own, and yet he accepts his new routine and has become a calmer child. His concentration span is also a lot longer.

We are now enjoying a very loving and affectionate child. My husband and I thank you most sincerely.

Research

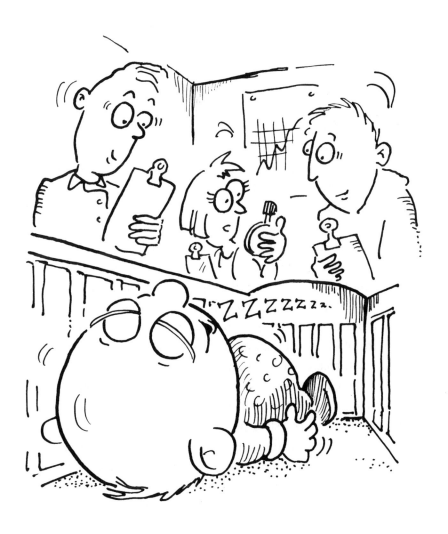

AN INTERESTING ASPECT of working in this area of child health is the amount of controversy which exists. Almost all new parents find that they are besieged with opinions from all sorts of people. Libraries and news-stands are generously endowed with publications giving advice and information. Unfortunately, many of these opinions contradict each other. Almost by definition, anybody who gives advice will find an opponent.

My training before I became a doctor was in science. Doctors are also trained in the scientific method and are taught to believe in the value of evidence. While the under-lying methods to improve sleep performance which I have been teaching for years were learned in the hot-house of parenthood and general practice consulting, I had always felt an obligation to subject the method to scientific analysis. This has recently been made possible with the generous support of the Research Foundation of the Womens and Childrens Hospital, Adelaide.

In the sleep literature there are a number of effective methods of improving sleep performance in children with sleep problems. The research literature is also very clear in showing how consistent and frequent sleep problems are in Western societies. Approximately 30 per cent of families will report some form of sleep disturbance in the first twelve months of the life of their infant that goes beyond the normal sleep disturbance of an infant feeding through the night.

My research aimed to test two things. The first was whether the protocol outlined in this book is useful. Does this method improve sleep performance in a measurable way? The second was whether the method is able to improve sleep performance in normal infants as opposed to infants who already have a sleep problem.

As mentioned above, there are many methods which have

been proven to improve sleep performance in children who have sleep problems. For many years, my style of consulting has focused on preventing the development of sleep disturbance by tutoring parents on sleep skills soon after their child is born. While this appeared to work in the clinical setting it needed to be scientifically proven or disproved.

A scientific study was designed in 1996 and run in 1997. The idea or hypothesis tested was that sleep performance in newborn infants could be improved by providing parents with tutoring in sleep theory from a research nurse and by giving them a copy of the first version of this book.

Three hundred and fifty families were recruited from birth notices in the public newspaper. Families were approached by telephone and offered participation in the trial. The trial was only open to normal infants with no major health problems. Once the family had agreed to participate they were divided randomly into two groups: the control group, and the intervention group.

The control group received no information or training from the sleep study. The intervention group received a tutorial from a trained research nurse within the first two weeks of life of their newborn infant. The tutorial lasted approximately 45 minutes and taught the key principles of sleep as outlined in this book. They were then provided with a copy of the previous edition of this book. The families were able to call the research nurse for assistance if they desired.

From the day the child reached six weeks of age and then again from the day the child reached twelve weeks, all the parents in both groups kept a sleep diary. This recorded the time of sleep, feeding, crying and waking achieved in twenty-four hour periods for seven consecutive days, with every hour divided into six ten-minute intervals. In total, 3200 days of data were collected and analysed.

In addition the parents' mood was studied by having them record a result on a depression score.

Results from the study were significant. By six weeks of age, infants in the intervention group, i.e. those whose parents had seen the research nurse and received a copy of the book, had achieved nine hours of additional sleep per week. This improvement in sleep performance was maintained at twelve weeks of age.

There is a statistical measure called a p value which is a measure of the chance that a particular scientific result has occurred by random error. For example, the chance of throwing a coin to show a head two times in a row is one-quarter or 0.25. The chance of throwing a head three times in a row is one-eighth or 0.125. The p value for the sleep study was less than one in a million. In other words, the chance is less than one in a million that the nine hours extra sleep in the intervention group compared to the control group was a result of random chance and not a result of improved sleep because of the protocol.

One of the potential criticisms of the method I teach is that it allows infants to cry on their own for long periods of time. The sleep diaries also recorded the length of time of crying. There was no difference between the control and the intervention groups in the total amount of crying recorded. These results were consistent at six weeks and twelve weeks of age.

As mentioned above, we also measured the mood score of the parents. The argument I had proposed was that if we were successful in showing improved sleep, and that was achieved, then the parents should have improved mood scores. Analysis of the results showed no significant difference between the two groups. Thus, even though the intervention group received an improved sleep this was not large enough to improve their emotions as measured by recording their self-assessment on a depression score.

One interesting finding was that the fathers in the study had slightly better mood scores than the mothers. This may reflect the general observation that mothers take a larger responsibility for the care of infants in the first months of life and are therefore more fatigued and more prone to depression and lower mood scores.

In conclusion, the study showed that the protocol outlined in this book is able to increase sleep performance by six weeks of age and that the improvement is maintained at twelve weeks. The average increase in sleep was nine hours per week. Most of this increased sleep occurred at night. There were no differences between the control and intervention group in total hours of crying. There was no significant improvement in the parents' mood score as a result of increased sleep.

Another area of controversy which I have faced over the years is the question of breast feeding. Those of you who have read the chapter on breast feeding will find that in certain circumstances I advocate the occasional use of a top-up bottle. This causes a great deal of anxiety among groups that advocate full breast feeding.

When I was practising as a country general practitioner, I decided to look at the use of top-up feeding by surveying 100 consecutive patients from our country hospital. All of these parents had been offered the use of top-up bottles while they were patients in hospital. At twelve weeks of age the infants were reviewed by telephone survey. The results were that 67 per cent of our patients were fully breast feeding. Of those who wished to breast feed, thus excluding those patients who had chosen to bottle feed from the time of birth of the baby, 75 per cent of mothers were fully breast feeding at twelve weeks. These results were compared to a study of 1100 infants carried out in South Australia in 1991. This larger study showed 53 per cent of women were fully breast feeding at twelve weeks. The p value for this, or the chance of the different result occurring by random error, was three chances in one thousand. This result suggests that the method advocated in this book appears to increase the chance of successful breast feeding and certainly not the reverse.

I have no doubt that debate will continue to occur in many areas of infant care. I have, to the best of my ability, checked, using a randomised controlled technique, that the protocol in this book is able to increase the number of hours sleep achieved without increasing the total amount of crying experienced by the baby. In addition the results of a retro-spective telephone survey suggest that there is an increased chance of successful breast feeding if a top-up bottle can be used on occasion.

I thank you for your attention. I hope very much that this book has been helpful and I wish you great joy in your children. Being a parent has been for me one of life's great rewards. Caring for many families with babies and young children and seeing their joy at achieving high quality sleep has been a privilege and brought me great satisfaction.

Appendix

Instant diagnosis

This appendix attempts to help parents to sort out some commonly observed behaviours. By its very nature it is simplistic and should be used as a guide only. If in doubt seek assistance from your medical adviser.

1 Baby crying

a Takes a feed well and then settles
- **hungry**

b Takes a feed poorly
Settles well in your arms
Unsettled in cot
- **overtired**

c Takes a feed poorly
Unsettled in cot
Unsettled in your arms
- **colic or other illness or very overtired**

d Taking feeds well or poorly

Bowels not open well

Hard pebbly bowel motions

- **constipation**

---

2 Feeding problems

---

a Feeds poorly at breast

Fails to sleep well

Settles in arms

Tearful

- **overtired**

---

b Feeding hungrily at breast

Becomes frustrated and angry

Rejects breast

Fails to settle

- **poor milk supply**

---

b Feeds well at breast

Spills frequently

Vomits after feed

Fails to settle

- **reflux**

---

d Feeds poorly at breast

Very sleepy

Poor weight gain

Few bowel actions

- **poor milk supply (needs help from your medical adviser quickly)**

---

3 Sleep disturbances

a Difficult to get to sleep

Woken by minor noises

Irritable

- **overtired**

b Constantly sleepy

Poor weight gain

Small hard irregular bowel action

- **undernourished (needs help from your medical adviser quickly)**

c Tearful late in day or after travelling

- **tired**

Index